"It is not the strongest of the species that survives, nor the most intelligent. It is the one that is most adaptable to change." - Charles Darwin (attributed)

"You try to plant a rose in the concrete, y'know what I mean? If it grow, and the rose petal got all kind of scratches and marks, you not gonna say, 'Damn, look at all the scratches and marks on the rose that grew from concrete'; you gonna be like, 'Damn! A rose grew from the concrete?!'" – Tupac Shakur

The
Kitchen Sink Farming
Series

Volume 1: Sprouting [Edition 1]

Publisher:
Stone Soup Publications
Portland, OR 97239

publisher@KitchenSinkFarming.org

In humble gratitude to the trees that grew to make the paper recycled to make this book. I've tried to use you wisely.

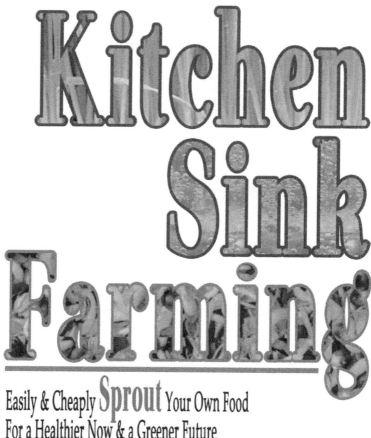

Kitchen Sink Farming

Easily & Cheaply Sprout Your Own Food
For a Healthier Now & a Greener Future

Volume 1
in the Kitchen Sink Farming Series

Jean-Pierre Parent

Also by Jean-Pierre Parent:

In the "Kitchen Sink Farming" Series:

- Vol 1: Sprouting
- Vol 2: Fermenting
- Vol 3: Growing
- Vol 4: Homegrown Living Recipes - What to Do with Your Sprouts and Krauts
- The Complete Set: All 4 Volumes

and

Practice Makes…Meditation and Yoga in Everyday Life

Jean-Pierre Parent's blogs

Food: www.KitchenSinkFarming.org

Yoga: www.OmInvasion.org

Contents

Preface

This book is the result of a serious personality flaw.

Somehow, from a very early age, I've rarely been satisfied with anything. Or, more accurately, I'm only satisfied with perfection, that acutely rare and delicate moment when the stars align; the air is just so, filling the lungs with sweet fortitude and the project before you sparkles with temporal rightness…

This eternal dissatisfaction with the lack of perfection pervades every aspect of my life: my athleticism, health, relationships, even conversations. I practice them beforehand, and I think about them afterwards, re-working them in my mind until my responses are the most thoughtful, compassionate, wise, and considerate statements possible.

As a little kid playing with my Atari, I hit the reset button on the console more often than the one on the controller, re-starting the game over and over if I did something that wasn't *quite* right, so that I could have another chance to do it again, only this time, perfectly. At the time, I think I expected all of life could be like that.

But I think I really hit my "always-satisfied-with-the-best" stride with food. If I was eating something (and that happened quite often in those days), I would wonder "what's the best possible form of this food?" So I cut out junk food and soda (I think I was nine at this time), after experiencing how I felt after eating a fast food hamburger before a soccer game. Didn't make that mistake again. I soon came to learn about vegetarian, then vegan, then organic, then raw food. The quest didn't stop there though, because of the widely varying ideas of raw vs. living food, organic standards, and genetic modification of food. Recently, the world's largest chain of natural food grocery stores was caught selling frozen vegetables as organic that were actually grown in China with little respect for chemical-free farming, and the "independent" organic certifiers that permitted the labeling are owned by the store (more on pg 27). So it's a constant question about who's trustworthy, and "how long will they be?" (See chapter "Truly Empty Calories", subchapter "When Organic Isn't (It's Too Easy Being Green)" for more on this particular paranoia).

Then there is the immeasurable question of taste. All this wholesome and nutritious food (much like the bland and boring natural choices offered when I was a kid, and 90% of them today) might be good for the body but unless it can create sublime waves of closed-eye, headed-tilted moaning pleasure, it does little for the soul. And therefore leaves something to be desired. Incomplete. Imperfect.

These days, my slightly mellowed aspirations for perfection have made me an experimenter, a scientist, a chef, a do-it-yourself-er. Before sitting down to write this (at a desk that I built so I could be the perfect height, with a pillow that I cut from the perfect density of memory foam mattress, on which I am sitting in a yoga position called siddhasana, or perfect pose), I noticed that some pumpkin seeds I sprouted and put in my dehydrator for a crunchy snack were sticking together. Makes sense, if you've ever lobotomized a pumpkin for a jack-o-lantern, scooping out its slimy stuck-

> "I have simple tastes. I am always satisfied with the best."
> – Oscar Wilde

together seeds. I thought that natural cohesion might be a good start to a flatbread, maybe mixed with super-sticky flax. So, did I make *a* pumpkinseed-flax flatbread? No... I made about 2 dozen. Equal parts flax and pumpkin. Double one, and double the other. Each one of those split in thirds, one part put on the counter to ferment, one in the oven at a low temp, and the rest in the dehydrator at a lower temp. Each of *those* split in half again, dry or with some oil. One in each category blended with some sprouted spelt, to see if they'd be better a little cake-ier. All labeled and catalogued. You get the idea.

Some may think that this level of precision is boring, rigid, anal-retentive, or obsessive, and I might agree if it was focused on a less important subject. But I think nourishment is just too important to be satisfied with anything less than utterly thorough knowledge, which until recently we've had to mostly figure out by our lonesomes. I think that this mindset is an integral part of being able to draw the measure of life's awesomeness and maybe the best way to experience the most happiness, fun, health, contentedness, and eventual freedom, because I will *know* what the best choice is for me today. With certainty. That's the goal, anyways. And then I'm happy, because the mundane turns into magic when it's dove into with attentive and receptive enthusiasm.

This book is the result of my decades-long experiment that asks the question: what's the best food possible, to fuel the best life possible? I think I've found glimmers of the answer, and I'm so pleased to be able to share them with you.

This is what led me to eating whole, organic, living foods: wanting to get as much out of my food as possible. Your reasons might be totally different. Starting with pure ingredients is a life-saver for someone with food allergies – the only way to take control of what goes into your body. Even someone lactose intolerant can enjoy the bowel-healing properties of milk (as raw kefir), butter (as ghee), or cheeses of many kinds (all in Kitchen Sink Farming Volume 2: Fermenting). Cancer patients find remission through fermented foods. The environmental benefits of enough home growers and sprouters will have a major global impact. A network of neighbors, each specializing in a different product could build a community like nothing else – focusing around the most primal and fundamental cement of society. And as I'll mention time and again, it's also the cheapest way to eat what is possibly the very best food in the world.

The "Why?"

The world's best foods aren't available in stores. You can't get them from the home shopping network, either. It's a good thing, too, because then people would buy them and miss out on the particular satisfaction of eating something they grew themselves, acutely aware of the life cycle of and organic rhythms of nature in their current mouthful. It's also a good thing because they're really cheap and really easy to make. Once you try it, it'd be laughable to pay someone else to do it. This book is based on the firm fact that anyone, anywhere, at any time, can be enjoying a bounty of fresh, living, incredibly nutritious food with very little work and expense.

Once you've enjoyed a delicious and vibrant lunch made from sprouted seeds, grains, or nuts bursting with taste and life, you won't need any convincing. You'll know by that point how easy, cheap, and fun it is to grow sweet strawberries, succulent micro greens, and juicy tomatoes with shocking depth of flavor in your seventh-story apartment kitchen, washing them down with home-brewed, wild-yeasted ginger ale or sparkling kombucha tea. In the meantime, though,

> "A great revolution in just one single individual will help achieve a *change* in the destiny of a society and, further, will enable a *change* in in the destiny of humankind."
> *Daisaku Ikeda*

before you figure all that out for yourself, it's supportive to know exactly why you're doing what you're doing. Maybe you're interested in increasing the amount of fresh, organic food you're eating (and there's no fresher food than something grown 5 feet away from your table and "picked" when you take your first chew!) and dramatically improving your health, energy, and immune system. Maybe you want to save money on groceries or have less of an impact on the earth, casting a vote against industrialized, destructive modern farming methods. Or maybe girls (and guys) just wanna have fun in the kitchen. Whatever your reason, learning about the myriad benefits of sprouting, indoor gardening, and fermenting at home will only encourage and inspire. And it just might make you able to explain to your mom why the dinner peas have leaves.

Nutrients and enzymes don't take kindly to cooking, canning, or sitting on shelves. Even fresh, organic produce loses valuable benefits every hour it's wilting away under the grocery store lights. In Los Angeles, it's hard to walk a few blocks and not pass a Whole Foods or organic restaurant. But even there, in the city with perhaps the greatest access to all things health, sprouted peanut butter, Kamut grass juice (wheat's superior ancestor), unpasteurized sauerkraut, enzymatically-active hot soups, and raw goat milk kefir are either not for sale, or else have to be painstakingly and expensively tracked down, even though they require very little knowledge, no expensive equipment, and less than a minute a day to make. When I was learning the things in this book, even though my efforts usually required a lot of trial and error, I kept coming back to the same eureka feeling: "It *can't* be this easy." But it is. A short and hopefully fun learning adventure will have you eating better than ever before, saving money, and feeling amazing. Maybe one day your local Piggly Wiggly will have a nut butter cafe, where they'll grind the freshly sprouted nuts of your choice, which you can spread on the apple a polite and well-groomed apron-clad deli worker just picked in front of you. If, and when we get there, through the slow and painstaking process of transforming consumer opinion and convincing the huge conglomerates that it's cost-effective to service us in this way, they'll surely charge an arm and a snout for it. No. The only way to eat living, vital, delicious food is to grow and prepare it yourself.

Nerd Corner!

Sprouting seeds increases their nutrient availability by 50-2000%, with an average of about 500%. See table on pages 14-15 to see the effects on specific nutrients after sprouting mung beans (not the most common spout, but possibly the most fun to say).

Nature is a hard-working and dedicated employee. Hire her to work for you and then sit back and relax. Nobody fertilizes or irrigates the forest. It's a complete system that does these things on its own. Make a "food forest" in your apartment, home, or patio, and your main effort is to pick the food. You put in some effort at the very beginning, but once the system is established, you work a lot less. You could call Kitchen Sink Farming "lazy agriculture", because you're working *with* nature, and not against her. You're using the laws of nature, forces that apply equally on a rainforest floor, a Brooklyn backyard, or a Tokyo high-rise to grow your lunch. Sprouting, fermenting, and growing your own food are plain and simply the best foods you can get. They require the least amount of energy to digest, contain the most nutrition, and have the least impact on the environment, resources, and humanity, providing for the longest, most disease and discomfort-free life. And wouldn't you know it: it's the cheapest and easiest way to create food, too. Anyone in the world can apply at least one principal in this book, and the more you work into your own everyday life, the better off that life will be for it.

Sprouting: Why Mess with a Perfectly Good Seed?

1) Sprouting activates enzymes.

Sprouts have an average of 7 times the number of enzymes needed to digest them, enzymes that can go to work digesting other foods, repairing and regenerating the body. See "Kitchen Sink Farming Vol 4: Homegrown Living Recipes - What to Do with Your Sprouts and Krauts" for more on enzymes.

> "Intelligence is the ability to adapt to change."
> Stephen Hawking

2) Sprouting Increases Nutrition.

Sprouted seeds supply nutrients in a predigested form – food is broken down into its simplest and easiest-to-digest components. During sprouting, much of the starch is broken down into simple sugars such as glucose and sucrose by the action of the enzyme 'amylase'. Proteins are converted into amino acids and amides. Fats and oils are converted into more simple fatty acids by the enzyme lipase. Sprouts are also high in fiber, so that along with their water content are even more helpful with digestion.

3) Sprouting Removes "Enzyme Inhibitors".

Enzyme Inhibitors keep seeds from sprouting at the wrong time, and keep nutrients locked up. Sprouting seeds also makes them easier to digest and more nutritious for this reason, actually making everything you eat before and after more nutritious too. (see pg 61 for more)

Table 1: Effects of Sprouting on Mung Beans

First two columns of chart reprinted from Critical Reviews in Food Science and Nutrition, 1989; 28(5):401-37. "Nutritional improvement of cereals by sprouting", Chavan JK, Kadam SS., Department of Biochemistry, Mahatma Phule Agricultural University, Rahuri, India.

Protein	Increases 30%	The increase in protein availability is an indicator of the overall enhancement of nutritional value of a sprouted seed.
Carbohydrates	Decreases 15%	The simultaneous reduction in carbohydrate and caloric content indicates that many carbohydrate molecules are broken down during sprouting to allow absorption of atmospheric nitrogen to reform it into amino acids. The resulting protein is the most easily digestible of all proteins.
Calcium	Increases 30%	
Potassium	Increases 80%	
Sodium	Increases 690%	The skyrocketing sodium content is a good indication that foods are much

		more easily digestible in the sprouted form, as sodium is essential to the digestive process, particularly in the intestines, and also to the elimination of carbon dioxide. The building blocks of both nutrition and digestibility peak simultaneously.
Iron	Increases 40%	
Vitamin A	Increases 285%	
Vitamin B1 (Thiamine)	Increases 208%	
Vitamin B2 (Riboflavin)	Increases 515%	
Vitamin B3 (Niacin)	Increases 256%	
Vitamin C	Infinite Increase	Dry seeds don't show a measurable amount of Vitamin C, but it skyrockets when they're sprouted. Vitamin C is important in the metabolization of proteins, which also increase in sprouted seeds.

A Deeper Reason to Take Control of Our Food: Truly Empty Calories

Food that's not organically grown by traditional, natural methods (paradoxically called "conventionally-grown") is fairly devoid of nutrients. Large-scale commercial farmers discovered in the 1940's that three nutrients are required to grow and produce normal-looking crops: nitrogen, phosphorous, and potassium, or NPK, but plants, like us, require over 100 minerals to be at their best, and if it's not in the soil, it's not on your plate. Plants grown "conventionally" don't have the nutrients they need to develop healthy immune systems, requiring farmers to spray them down with a heavy coat of pesticides, herbicides, and fungicides. When we eat the fruit and vegetables that come off of nutrient-deficient, chemical pesticide-laden plants, we suffer in two ways: very little nutrition and a dose of cancer-causing chemicals. When I'm travelling and can't get organic produce, I feel as if I'm eating photographs of food. The apples look like apples, they're red and round, but they're tasteless and my body feels a lifeless chunk of food in my belly as if I've been chewing on paper. My body is waiting for the flood of nourished happiness that it's used to, but doesn't come.

It gets worse. Turns out this disconnect is the well-planned stratagem of big business, that can almost always be counted on to put profits before people. Consumers are starting to become aware of a decades-old curtain of misinformation and propaganda drawn between grocery store shoppers and the contents of their carts by

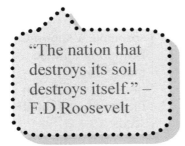

"The nation that destroys its soil destroys itself." – F.D.Roosevelt

massive agribusiness and its bigger, cheaper, faster business model. But it wasn't always this way.

A History of Agri-Tech

Before World War II, people farmed the way they always have: fertilizing their fields with nutrient-dense organic matter or growing where rivers overflow and deposit the year's worth of mineral-rich silt. They rotated crops so plants that take certain nutrients from the soil are supported by a

> "Humanity consumed 120% of the earth's sustainable resource capacity in 1999" - National Academy of Sciences, June 2007

season of plants that put those nutrients back. They relied on the strength of the crops' own immunity to fight off pests. Rainbows glittered over every dew-speckled family-farmed field of organic heirloom veggies... Ok, not really, but food *was* more nutritious and less carcinogenic.

World War II inspired many advances in industrial science, from napalm and synthetic rubber to the atomic bomb. When it was over, huge stocks of nitrates from ammunition building, organophosphates for making nerve gas, and other chemicals had accumulated. Nitrates contain nitrogen, one component of the NPK triad, and an enterprising chemical company re-labeled them "fertilizer". Nerve agents like mustard gas, shown to block communication between the brain and organs in both humans and insects alike, were called "pesticides", and both of these were sold to post-war farms. These chemicals, with only slight variations are still used today, and over 1.5 million pounds of organophosphates are sprayed every year on California farms alone.

The huge demand placed on modern farmers to feed more and more people on less and less space is creating an unparalleled desperation. In an attempt to keep up with demand, farmers have fired nature and are courting the promise of a dangerous and only partially-understood technology.

Burger & a Side of Flies: Genetic Modification of Food

Pick a single-ingredient food off the supermarket shelves and you have a 70% chance of grabbing a genetically modified organism, or GMO. This is the volatile and very scary process of splicing a fruit, veggie, or grain's DNA with genes from another organism, always part bacteria, often animal and sometimes even insect, human, or virus. Choose something with corn (or a derivative like corn syrup, dextrose, baking powder, caramel and caramel coloring, mono and diglycerides, modified food starch, vegetable anything: broth, oil, protein, shortening, and the many other ways industrious food scientists have found to pump the most heavily-subsidized and therefore most commonly-grown crop in the US into our diets) or a food with more than a few ingredients and unless it's organic or specifically labeled "non-GMO", your chances of choosing a genetically modified organism go up to around 100%. The ancient process of plant breeding is this: put two plants with traits you like next to each other and hope they'll cross-pollinate and the next generation will be an even better plant.

This wasn't precise or fast enough for modern agribusiness. GMO was born out of the desire to achieve total dominion over crops, under the guise of lowering costs and increasing yields. But as with the attempt to control most things in nature, the outcome was not the expected one. Genetic modification has actually cost agriculture more, after recalls on untamable seeds, the inability of GM plants to access nutrients in the soil, puzzlingly lower yields in drought conditions and increased needs for more powerful pesticides with the consequence of mutant super-weeds. None of these issues have impeded cell-invasive technology's expansion, however, as the planting of GM crops went from zero acres in 1988 to 3.7 million in 1996 to 100 million in 2003. Most of the financial burden has fallen not on the slick-talking companies, however, but on the farmers who were taken in by their glimmering promises. It becomes a deadly gamble when, like between 2001 and 2005, 32,000 Indian farmers committed suicide underneath the avalanche of debt an Indian subsidiary of the Monsanto Corporation pawned off onto them when their GM cotton fields were ravaged by a disease that affected only GM plants. Ironically, at least one of the farmers killed himself, at 25 years old, by drinking a liter of pesticide.

Monsanto is one of the companies that is single-handedly destroying the traditional methods of farming in favor of a near-fascist domination of farmers and the very DNA of the seeds they plant, and along with it the worlds' food supply. Monsanto, whose first success was Agent Orange, the forest defoliant used in the Vietnam War are and has since been found guilty in Federal courts of falsifying their earnings statements (Foreign Corrupt Practices Act (15 U.S.C. § 78dd-1)), bribing government officials around the globe (15 U.S.C § 78m(b)(2) & (5)), knowingly polluting the small town of Anniston, Alabama, with dangerous levels of polychlorinated biphenyls (PCBs) resulting in over 3.500 cases of cancer and other degenerative diseases, mislabeling pesticides to minimize their dangers (*Monsanto guilty of chemical poisoning in France*, Reuters Feb 13, 2012) and countless other crimes against humankind and nature. In the year 2000, it was estimated that 10 new people everyday are diagnosed with cancer due to exposure to dioxin produced by Monsanto (US Environmental Protection Agency's (EPA) draft reassessment on dioxin) and as of this writing, Monsanto is being taken to court by a group of Argentinean tobacco farmers who say that the biotech giant knowingly poisoned them with herbicides and pesticides and subsequently caused "devastating birth defects" in their children.

But the *really* scary part of this whole mess is that these "franken-foods" reproduce in unexpected and uncontrollable ways. Bizarre monstrosities of barely recognizable plants discovered in fields. 1000-generational heirloom corn farms contaminated by invading mutant DNA. Monsanto's BT corn, cotton, and soy are *themselves*

"A molecular study conducted by Mexican, American and Dutch researchers demonstrates the presence of genes from genetically modified organisms (GMO) among the varieties of traditional corn cultivated in the remote regions of Oaxaca State in the southern part of the country, even though the Mexican government has always maintained a moratorium on the use of transgenic seed." - from "GMO Contamination in Mexico's Cradle of Corn" *Le Monde*, December 11 2008

registered as pesticides. The process of genetically modifying foods is not only unethical and disgusting, but we're messing with forces we don't understand and the current results are hinting at world-wide epidemics of sci-fi horror film proportions. For example, in 1989 there was an outbreak of a new disease in the US, traced back to a batch of an L-tryptophan food supplement produced with GMO bacteria. Though it contained less than .1% of the highly toxic compound, 37 people died that year and 1,500 were left with permanent disabilities.

The Food and Drug Administration declared that it was not gene modification that was at fault but a failure in the purification process. However, the company concerned, Showa Denko, admitted that the low-level purification process had been used without ill effect in non-GM batches. Scientists at Showa Denko blame the GM process for producing traces of a potent new toxin, and this new toxin had never been found in non-GM versions of the product. In May 2008, new findings by the Physicians and Scientists for Responsible Application of Science and Technology (PSRAST) caused them to state, "Most importantly, the poison considered most important in the tryptophan was closely similar to

"Typically, if something is to be considered Generally Recognized as Safe (G.R.A.S.) it needs lots of peer-reviewed published studies and an overwhelming consensus among the scientific community. With GM crops, they had neither." – Jeffrey Smith, author, *Seeds of Deception*

tryptophan (a dimer), but never found in natural bacteria. This indicates that disturbed tryptophan metabolism generated the poison. Moreover, the inserted genes were directed at altering the metabolism (so as to increase tryptophan production).

Our conclusion is that the only plausible explanation for the appearance of this poison is disturbances of the natural metabolic processes due to genetic engineering."

This is just one example of the dangers of genetic manipulation. It's easy to imagine that every instance of genetic modification has its own tale, or will. In fact, children have more adverse reactions to GMOs than adults, and it's hard to not picture a future without horrible consequences from freely fucking with nature.

From news footage of Vice President George Bush Sr. at the Monsanto factory in 1987:

Monsanto Executive: "We have no complaint about the way the USDA is handling it; they're going through an orderly process… Now if we're waiting til September and we don't have our authorization we may say something different!"

Bush: "Call me. We're in the de-reg [de-regulation] business. Maybe we can help."

The idea hits home even harder when a public official in Japan, where GM foods are outlawed stated their plan to "watch US children for the next ten years" before they determine their next course of action, according to the documentary "The Future of Food" (Deborah Koons Garcia, Lily Films, 2004).

Bio-engineered foods don't have, and were never designed, to provide any benefit to the consumer. No attempt has been made to make more nutritious wheat or better-tasting spinach. Instead, the GM industry's only goal is profit (of everyone but the farmer), so the scam has been sold to the American consumer as a way to provide food for the masses of overpopulated future generations. One problem with this logic is that the nearly 1 billion malnourished people (10,000 of which die every day from starvation) don't do so because of a lack of food. Many of these people used to be farmers, but were kicked off their land when their respective governments accepted huge loans from multi-national banks, and subsistence farming wasn't a workable way to pay them back. Forced off their farms and into the slums of industrializing third-world cities, they have gone from being food independent to food-dependant. The calamitous issue of world hunger is not a problem of production; it's a crisis of access, which is strange when one considers that the average piece of food travels 1500 miles from the farm to the supermarket. The other argument with this propaganda is Monsanto's plan to include in all seeds they produce a "terminator gene", a self-destructing abomination that creates a plant with sterile progeny. That means that if you buy a seed from Monsanto and plant it, instead of being able to harvest the seeds from your plants for next year, you will have to buy more seeds. This is clear proof that the biotech industry has no interest in "feeding the world", as their propaganda states. In the same way that GMO seeds have mysteriously found their

20

way into native plant genes (see quote below), the danger of this terminator gene out-crossing into the plants that make up the world's food supply, effectively ending traditional, sustainable farming, must have gone unnoticed by the company's scientists and members of the USDA who both approved the use of the gene and co-own it. No one can be that evil.

But who is responsible if terminator genes cross-contaminate unsuspecting food supplies? By past precedent, it's not the seed company that's to blame but the farmer, and courts have told farmers that by not protecting their fields properly from seeds blowing in (an absolutely ludicrous idea), they have unwittingly signed a contract with the biotech company that's patented that specific invading gene. Is it possible that one day the world's entire food supply will be controlled by the company that brought us PCB's (which are present in the cells of every man, woman, and child on Earth), DDT, bovine growth hormone, and dioxins, and who has bribed government officials to look the other way while illegally dumping 50 tons of mercury into one Alabama river, stating "We cannot afford to lose one dollar of business", in an internal memo (a leaked copy of which is readily available online) found when this criminal polluting was exposed?

"AG Biotech will find a supporter occupying the White House next year, regardless of which candidate wins the election in November." – Monsanto In-House Newsletter, Oct 6, 2000, in reference to the multiple White House officials that are also board members of Monsanto.

Monsanto does, however, have most

of America's, and soon the world's, farmers completely dependent on them each planting season. And their wrath is swift and brutal against farmers even suspected of saving viable seeds. Even farmers with neighboring fields that have had these manipulated genes carried by the wind into their crops, which then cross into the genes of the new plants, are pressured with debilitating lawsuits to either go out-of-business or sign a contract and enter into the cycle of dependence and perversion.

Not surprisingly, by current FDA regulations, GMO foods aren't allowed to be labeled as such.

"We received over 44,000 pages from the FDA's own files and they revealed that the FDA has been lying to the world since 1992, if not before. But they continue to lie, they're still lying, they claim that there's an overwhelming consensus in the scientific community that genetically engineered foods are as safe as their conventionally produced counterparts and they claim that there has been sufficient data to back up this consensus. [Based on the FDA files] both of those claims are blatant lies." Steven Druker, lawyer for the Alliance for Bio-Integrity, who forced the FDA to unclassify its internal files on GMOs.

And back to the history... After WWII, famers began growing just one crop on a field, requiring more and more chemical support as the malnourished plants weakened. In fact, according to the National Resources Defense Council, pesticide use since the 1940's has gone up 10 times, but crop loss due to insects has doubled, and in the meantime, the Environmental Protection Agency estimates that there are pesticide residuals in the tissues of every American. Our current agricultural system now relies on toxic fertilizers to keep the land producing food, as the precious topsoil that took thousands of years to develop is being washed away at an

"This [genetic modification of food] is the largest biological experiment humanity has ever entered into." – Dr. Ignacio Chapel, Microbial Biologist, UC Berkeley

alarming rate. In fact, in the last 50 years, America has lost over 75% of its fertile soil. It takes 200 to 1000 years to create just one inch of topsoil; no modern technology can make it faster than that. Add to that the fact that the world's main food-producing countries like the US, China, India, Australia and Spain have or are about to reach their water resource limits, and you have an unsustainable agricultural system that can't go on this way much longer. Our dependence on chemical agriculture is a slippery slope. Like hard drugs, we need more and more to get the same effects. Something's gotta give, or soon there will be no seeds to sow, no topsoil to sow them in, no water to water them with, and certainly no way to protect them from the very gentlest of bugs. The only way out is for you and me to take responsibility for what we're putting into our bodies by growing it ourselves, not just voting for change but passionately and peacefully dissenting against an untenable system by planting or sprouting a seed and eating it with delight.

There is hope that the US will follow the example of Europe and Japan who, not beholden to the rebates, subsidies, and political and collegiate contributions of the biotech industries, have outlawed all GM foods. A federal judge recently invalidated the patent on a gene that is known to cause breast cancer, owned by Myriad Genetics in association with the University of Utah, who charged exorbitant fees to research facilities using the gene to research breast cancer prevention. This ruling casts doubt on the motives of the companies holding gene patents and raises important ethical questions about the ability to patent life.

When Organic Isn't (It's too easy being green)

Obviously, it's better to buy organic food over conventional. It's a vote for the health of your family, your community, and the environment. Unfortunately, just choosing produce with an organic sticker isn't enough. I want to believe the strict and stringent guidelines for organic certification are followed by

"If we're still dragging our feet in 2015, it really becomes almost impossible for the world to avert a degree of climate change that we simply will not be able to manage", John Holdren, Professor of Environmental Policy, Harvard University, and Director of the White House Office of Science and Technology Policy

participating farms with enthusiasm and far-sighted wisdom, but I know too much about the funding the certifiers receive from the corporations whose goal it is to relax the laws for the betterment of their immediate profits. I hear too many stories from friends in the biz who are told to slap an organic sticker on every fifth crate of asparagus they're packing and call it a day. In 2005 in the UK, the widespread epidemic of fraudulently labeling meat as organic was a scandal that required a major government crackdown. The USDA, America's main certification agency who both makes the rules and sells organic certification, is heavily funded by Monsanto and other biotech conglomerates. It's companies like these that are fighting for (and paying for) more lenient rules within an increasingly lucrative market.

And it's working: a 2006 amendment created a list of 38 synthetic ingredients allowed in products that can still be called organic. This allowed Anheuser-Busch in 2007 to have its "Wild Hop Lager" certified organic even though it uses hops grown with chemical fertilizers and sprayed with pesticides. Advocacy groups fear that, since almost all organic foods are now sold through high-volume distribution channels like Target and Wal-Mart (the #1 retailer of organics in the US), the laws will change to support the massive producers, and the small farms that pioneered traditional methods of farming will be squeezed out. While they wait for the laws to change, Wal-Mart continually pressures their suppliers to cut corners, if not to break laws outright. In 2007, Aurora Organic Dairy, Wal-Mart's main supplier of organic dairy products, was found to be in violation of 14 organic regulations and would have lost their certification if it weren't for some unusual leniency on the part of the FDA. The truth is, the organic label can be bought, and is at best a vague indication of standards practiced in fields and facilities. On the other side of the coin, many small farms that operate according to organic guidelines and beyond aren't certified simply because they can't afford to be.

The simple truth is that big business cannot be trusted to do the right thing when millions or billions of dollars are at stake. Advertisers use buzz words like "fresh", "family-owned", "natural", or "local", not in an effort to accurately describe, but to sell with little interest in the truth. It's gotten quite out of hand how advertisers can say absolutely anything and we, in our nose-to-the-grindstone haste to feel better, or check "good for us" off of our grocery lists, let ourselves be unthinkingly swayed.

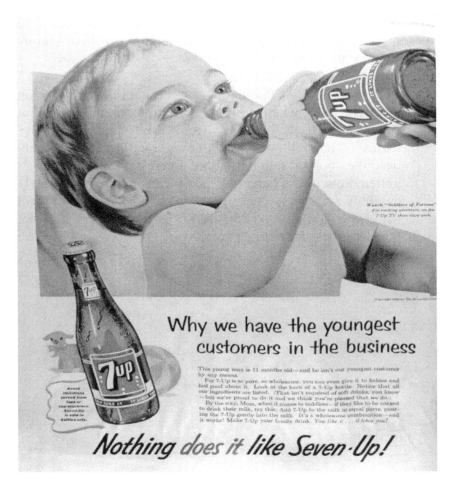

A would-be-funny-if-it-wasn't-so-sad example of deceptive 1955 advertising. Will we look back in 50 years with an equally ironic sophistication to Wendy's "You Know When It's Real" campaign, Nestle's "eco-shaped bottled water", and the other 98% of products world-wide tested in 2009 (by TerraChoice, who runs the Environmental Choice Program *for the Canadian government) whose labels were found to be misleadingly green-washed?*

Recently, the world's largest chain of natural food grocery stores came under fire for misrepresenting the quality of their store-brand frozen organic vegetables. Turns out the "Organic California Blend", as well as snap peas, spinach, and some others, were produced in China, and the store misleadingly and illegally put "USDA Organic" and "QAI" (Quality Assurance International) stamps on the foods, though neither organization had inspected the farms or food. They have, however, inspected hundreds of tons of food grown in China that were contaminated with chemicals and/or pathogens.

These stories shed light on the dark corners of the entire organic movement, which retailers like Whole Foods have ridden to massive financial success. Agriculture giants like Gerber's, Heinz, *Dole*, ConAgra and ADM, who have no problem poisoning workers, consumers, and the Earth with toxic chemical practices have jumped on the bandwagon with Earthy-friendly sounding organic subsidiaries. It takes little common sense to realize that

"If people let government decide what foods they eat, their bodies will soon be in as sorry a state as are the souls of those who live under tyranny." –Thomas Jefferson

massive conglomerates, who commonly purchase pesticides that have been outlawed in the US to use in their South American plants before shipping them back to American consumers (a bizarre loophole in the law), can't be trusted to make ethical decisions about my food when one simple lie can net them millions of dollars. Same goes for Target, recently sued for mislabeling natural products like rice milk and tofu as organic. Or that, though "organic farm" and "small family farm" are interchangeable in most consumers' minds, almost all the organic food produced in America comes from California, where 5 or 6 huge operations dominate the market. 80% of US beef is produced by 4 companies[1]. The vast majority of the seeds planted by the world's farmers come from 4 conglomerations of companies. Food retailers are also on a consolidation track. By some estimates, within the next ten years all of the retail food in the world will be controlled by 6 companies, only one of which will be American, Wal-Mart. Represent! This means that the selection and labeling of products on your grocery store shelves will be decided by a broker, potentially on another continent, based on what will return the largest profit.

If you sprout and grow your own food, you know it's organic. If you buy it, you only hope it is.

Home growing, sprouting, and fermenting is one of the best ways to take responsibility for your own health and impact on the environment, and creates a haven from the conspiracy of corporate greed and consumer manipulation that plays like a Hollywood movie. The few seconds it takes to rinse our sprouts can re-establish our primordial bond to the land, the elements, and the moment-to-moment birth, maturation, and transformation of the pulsating forces

---

[1] Nebraska and S Dakota passed constitutional amendments banning all farms not family-owned. Corporate agri-business didn't like that one bit, but state constitutions (and government in general) are in fact of, by, and for the people. Oops.

of life around us. Even 100 glass and steel stories above the cement, life presses powerfully on. All this from an unused square-foot spot on a kitchen counter or closet shelf that would otherwise be collecting dust or worse, historical spoons from ebay.

Collapse, the Future of Food

"A living planet is a much more complex metaphor for deity than just a bigger father with a bigger fist. If an omniscient, all-powerful Dad ignores your prayers, it's taken personally. Hear only silence long enough, and you start wondering about his power. His fairness. His very existence. But if a world mother doesn't reply, Her excuse is simple. She never claimed conceited omnipotence. She has countless others clinging to her apron strings, including myriad species unable to speak for themselves. To Her elder offspring She says – 'Go raid the fridge. Go play outside. Go get a job. Or, better yet, lend me a hand. I have no time for idle whining.'" - David Brin, physicist and sci-fi writer

At a certain point, the rate of global extraction of crude petroleum products is reached, after which the rate of production enters a terminal decline. This is called "Peak Oil" and is another reason to become self-sustainable sooner than later. This is to say that there will come a day when our oil use will surpass the oil that's left in the ground, heading us towards the inevitable moment when there's no more left to power our cars and homes, our electric plants, to make our fertilizers and pesticides, or to run our farm equipment, or the trucks that bring us the food.

Let's talk again about how commercial farms work. A field is fertilized, and all commercial fertilizers are made from ammonium nitrate, which is made from natural gas. This is sprayed onto the fields by an oil-powered machine. Another oil-powered machine ploughs and another comes by and plants. The fields are irrigated with pumps powered by electricity, which comes from coal or, you guessed it: natural gas. But wait, there's more - oil-powered crop dusters spray oil-derived pesticides, once, twice, thrice. Then, when it's time to harvest, one oil-powered machine cuts, another loads, and another takes it to where it'll be processed by electric contraptions, and it's wrapped in plastic (made of oil) and trucked to a distribution center, then to the store. You can take it from there. There are 10 calories of hydrocarbon energy in every one calorie of food produced this way. Imagine that there's a finite amount of oil in the world and you'll soon realize that this would be a blatantly unsustainable system. Unfortunately, we'll soon be forced to see the end of this strategy.

Oil is made from the fossilized bodies of microorganisms, a process that takes millions of years. As of this writing, half of all the oil in the world has been used. The remaining half is of increasingly lower quality and will require more and more

"Our agriculture system is almost wholly dependent on cheap fuel. Tremendous amounts of diesel fuel that are used in planting, and harvesting, and then, moving the stuff all these vast distances." - James Howard Kunstler *The Long Emergency*

energy to extract and refine. Oil is finite. Natural gas is finite, coal, uranium; all non-renewable energy sources are finite. There will be a peak for all of them. We're using, in a few decades, energy resources that took the planet millions of years to produce. Right now we are consuming 5 barrels of oil for every 1 barrel discovered.

For as long as I can remember, just about everyone I knew consumed like there was no tomorrow. My family threw away more food than many families in developing countries had. Now, when some of us in the West are just beginning to wake up to the realities of our wasteful lifestyle choices, those that have looked on hungrily for decades are starting to be able to enjoy the ease and luxury of modern life. In 1993, China had three quarters of a million cars on the road. At the start of 2004 they had 6 million, and now (2010) they have 24 million. The idea behind a "developing" country is that one day they'll be able to consume like a first world country; they'll be able to live like the people in the movies. But this is clearly impossible. Even Americans in the near future won't be able to consume like Americans today.

Most of us have our heads in the sand about this to one degree or another; we know there's a problem looming but we're hoping that if we bring our own bags to the supermarket it'll go away. But the average person in a developed country can't really be blamed; with the demands of modern life, most people are happy with just a few minutes a day to relax and enjoy the life they're working so hard for. We've never had a peak in resources before and we have blinders on about it. Like statistics about climate change or overpopulation on a piece of paper, it's not an idea we can easily digest. We need new role models.

Peak Oil Pioneers

From 1950 to 1990, Cuba lived comfortably under Soviet communist care. Then, with little warning in 1991, the Soviet Union collapsed and Cuba's access to oil dropped to less than 25%. Everything changed in a matter of weeks. Suddenly, malnourished children, anemic pregnant women, and underweight babies became commonplace. The impact on food production and availability was disastrous. The average Cuban lost 20 pounds. Massive blackouts made refrigeration difficult so the little food that was available would often spoil. Cubans had to wait 3 to 4 hours for a bus to take them to school or work, and when it came it was often full, so they'd have to wait another 3 to 4 for the next one. And when they finally got to work, there might be no power, or no materials for them to do their jobs.

Then in 1992, the 30-year-old American embargo of Cuba was tightened. Before, companies were prohibited from doing business with both communist Cuba and the freedom-defending USA. Now, any ship even docking in a Cuban port was denied access to the US for 6 months afterwards. Almost overnight, 750 million dollars worth of food and medical supplies pulled up

"So we had now been like an experiment, with controlled conditions… Nothing, or very little… could get in from the outside, so everything had to happen from the inside. " - Roberto Perez, Cuban permaculturist and educator, from documentary film *The Power of Community*

anchor and sailed away. Then in 1996, the stranglehold was intensified. Cuba abruptly found itself with almost no access to foreign resources. The American dollar was worth 150 pesos, and the average daily salary was worth 20 pesos. Cubans were making about 4 dollars a month, so money was no longer a commodity that could be used to acquire the basics of life. A recently comfortable society abruptly found itself cut-off, destitute, and hungry.

Every aspect of Cuban life was affected, but none more potently than farming. Before the collapse, Cuba's agriculture was more industrialized than any other Latin American country. It used a massive amount of fossil fuel for fertilizer, pesticides, farm machinery, and transportation - 2 or 3 times more than any other Latin American country, and acre for acre it surpassed the US in fertilizer consumption. Their farms had high yields, but these were in huge single-crop operations like tobacco, sugarcane, and citrus, which were exported while the basics were imported. The system wasn't set up to feed the people.

So the people: doctors, engineers, and lawyers, started sowing seeds in open places, without knowing how, because they were starving and there was no end in sight. The older generation, those that remembered how to operate a plough, how to tell if soil was acidic or alkaline by rolling it around in their mouths, were suddenly a valuable resource. A movement to use every arable piece of local land for growing food began. Every park, front yard, school, and vacant lot in Havana became a garden or orchard because there was no gas to transport food. And because there were no fossil fuels to produce chemical pesticides and fertilizers, over the months and seasons the fledgling farmers learned to use natural, organic pesticides like bugs and companion plants. Organic fertilizers like manure and compost were all they had.

They found ways to replenish the depleted soil with cheap and available resources, and to do their farming without the use of machinery. They used worms to turn sandy, dead soil into lush and nutrient-rich fertile ground. They found that they could extend the growing season by putting a fiber mesh between the plants and the sun, which would also control pests and was easily replaceable during hurricane season. As time went on, Cuban urban farmers found infinite small solutions to improve their lives. They dealt with the myriad complex problems that come with a new kind of agronomy by trial and error, and thrived. Formerly larger farms were divided up and leased to citizens for free by the government and the 2.2 million residents of Havana fed themselves from these rooftop gardens, schoolyard nurseries, and small farms within a few kilometers from the city.

Today, urban gardens in small Cuban cities and towns are even more productive, providing 80-100% of the residents' food, and over 80% of Cuba's food production is organic. In the 1980's, Cuba used 21,000 tons of chemical pesticides per year; now they use less than 1000. Good for the soil, good for the environment, good for the economy, and great for the people.

Now, apartment-dwellers with a well laid-out porch, rooftop, or patio garden improve their lives by both cutting back on their food-spending and selling their produce or homemade products like wine. Cuba's 140,000 urban farmers aren't the poorest people in society, as they are in many countries, like America, where farmers are constantly forced to cut corners and take the chemical way out. They are among the highest-paid professionals in the country, and are even exporting their natural pesticides, fertilizers, and knowledge to other countries. This rewarding occupation attracts people from all walks of life who don't want to be dependent on others for their sustenance. They have the respect of their communities and dignity of working in what has become one of the noblest professions.

The country as a whole is enjoying a slew of fringe benefits as well. They developed bio-organic farming methods because at the time they had no other choice. But now, with less than 2% of the population of Latin America, Cuba has 11% of its scientists. At the start of the "Special Period", the name for Cuba's quiet revolution starting with the collapse of the Soviet Union, Cuba had 3 universities. It now has about 50, with 7 in Havana alone. Cuba's urban farmers produce much more from the same amount of land than their corporate counterparts, and many of them donate a portion of their crops to the elderly, day-care centers and schools, orphanages, and pregnant women. They do this for free with no government involvement, because they want their community to thrive. Small farmers form co-ops, if they wish, to buy in bulk and share machinery. In many cities in richer countries, we don't even *know* our neighbors.

"It wasn't the *Exxon Valdez* captain's driving that caused the Alaskan oil spill. It was yours." - Greenpeace advertisement, 1990

Cuba has roughly the same life expectancy and infant mortality rate as the US, though the average citizen uses 1/8th the energy and resources of the average American. They were once forced to be frugal with their energy consumption, using the sun to pre-heat cooking water, for example, but now it's a way of life. Why do most American homes have their hot-water heaters in cold closets and basements, requiring more fossil fuels to heat them, instead of outside in the sun? Sugar mills, which produce gas when the fibers are heated, are used as power plants, which now provide the country with 30% of its energy during harvest seasons. Increased walking and biking improved Cubans' fitness and drastically reduced diabetes (51% less deaths attributed to diabetes since before the Soviet collapse), heart disease (35% less), and strokes (20% less, and 18% less deaths overall). Cuba trains more doctors than they need, more than double the number of physician-to-citizen ration as America, and sends the surplus to developing countries around the world. Urban planners from all over the world study Havana as a model of livability. 85% of Cubans own their own home. The countryside, which has been called the last romantic place on earth, looks like a science-fiction comic book come alive with solar cell home-spun shacks, country school and rural hospitals. Cuba has reclaimed its health, its communities, its ethos, and its future.

The fact that Cuba is still looking for oil off their shores may surprise some. But unlike the vampires in developed countries that will start wars and enslave weaker nations for the life-blood of their consumer culture, they don't use what they find. If Cuba does hit upon the Texas tea, they sell it to wealthier countries at a premium, because they know how to get by without it. We can wait until our own energy crisis to enact sustainable practices, and certainly the GOP government and their "head in the sand" policy-making will wait until it's too late, or we can make changes now while we have some breathing room.

The concept of peak oil brings up another, much bigger question: what will happen to us when the greasy lubricant of our society becomes too expensive to be a viable means of energy?

Easter Island's Last Lumberjack

Easter Island is a remote dot of earth about 1500 miles off the coast of Chile. It's so small you can walk around the whole thing in a day. It's also the hauntingly desolate remains of a once-thriving civilization that numbered over 10,000 people.

> "There is a sufficiency in the world for man's need but not for man's greed." – Mahatma Gandhi

When Easter Island was settled by 20 or 30 Polynesians halfway through the first millennium, it was a lush forest. The sweet potatoes and other crops the settlers brought with them thrived in the rich soil, living was easy, and the Easter Islanders found themselves with lots of free time. In about 1000 years, they swelled to a burgeoning society, and one of the most technologically advanced in the ancient world. Crops were protected by complex rock formations, and by some accounts every rock on the island was moved at least 3 or 4 times. The island's famous 600 stone statues, many of which were in sophisticated astronomical alignment, weighed tens of tons and were transported by human force, often for several miles over forested, hilly terrain. Each monument was laboriously carved from different color rock from quarries all over the island so the leaders of the clans could ask for favors from the Gods, and for a while it seemed to be working. But when European explorers reached the island in 1722, they found an arid grassland with less than 2000 malnourished people, many of who had become cannibals, living in squalid reed huts and constant warfare. The explorers couldn't fathom how such a primitive society could be responsible for the socially and technologically advanced monuments, and because the island was now a barren prairie, the transportation of behemoth idols seemed impossible. When asked how the 20-foot-high stone gods had gotten there, the inhabitants, wholly disconnected from their history, replied simply, "They walked".

Actually, the statues were pushed along rolling roads made of the island's trees, chopped down in huge swathes to make way for the huge stone carvings and laid side-by-side through miles of forest. The trees, which provided shelter, canoes for fishing, and fuel, were so abundant at the time that they could be used without fear of running out. But as the population continued to swell, and more and more clans were formed with more leaders, all needed their own statues lest their dependants miss out on their slice of the divine benevolence pie and the ability to live as well as their neighbors. Competition for resources between clans grew fierce, and then someone, one day, cut down the last tree on the island. No more boats for fishing. No more fuel for heat, cooking, or transporting statues. The topsoil eroded at a breakneck pace and the gravely land couldn't hold in moisture or nutrients. Hundreds of great stone deities were abandoned, unfinished, in quarries around the islands. The gods were not happy. With no logs for buildings, people began living in caves and flimsy reed huts, fiercely protecting their meager assets. Cannibalism became a reasonable means of dealing with both enemies and hunger. Like the Romans, Byzantines, Vikings, and Mayans before them, the Easter Islanders didn't think total collapse could happen to them, and lived recklessly until it did.

The pattern is clear. When civilizations over-consume, they cut off the legs of their own life-support systems and begin to fight each other over what little is left. Then they either starve or leave. Our current problems are global: climate change, overpopulation, peak oil, genetically manipulated genes out-crossing into the DNA of the world's food supply; so there's nowhere to go, just like boatless Easter Islanders on a remote island in the middle of the Pacific. We can't abandon our planet and set off for a new Eden. We're here, and we have only two choices: cut down the last tree, or take an objective look at the dilemmas facing our species as a whole, and find another way to live.

> "We never know the worth of water till the well is dry." - Thomas Fuller, *Gnomologia*, 1732

A very early action of the Bush administration upon assuming office in 2001 was to lobby for the replacement of the chairman of the official United Nations Intergovernmental Panel on Climate Change (IPCC). This was done at the request of Exxon, who felt the sitting chairman, Dr. Watson, was too "aggressive" in pursuing action on the issue of global warming. As a result of actions taken by the administration, Dr. Watson was replaced ("at the request of the US") by the industry-friendly Dr. Rajendra Pachauri, hand-picked by the administration, and referred to by former vice-president Al Gore as the "let's drag our feet" candidate. Four years later, Dr. Pachauri issued the strongest warning yet in regard to global climate change, and a most urgent call for immediate action. His report stated that there is not a moment to lose, and added that we are risking the ability of the human race to survive. He called for "very deep" cuts in current pollution levels, stating that the point of no return was rapidly approaching.

"The American way of life is non-negotiable" - Dick Cheney

Sometimes big change comes through a big effort. But more often, revolution is the result of very small actions repeated over time. For a while, maybe for several generations, the results of our efforts are almost unnoticeable, but then there comes a "tipping point" where the slow incremental change has completely reshaped society. It's like driving. Turn the wheel dramatically and you find yourself on the beginning of a different road, or in a ditch. But turn the wheel just 5 degrees, and for a while it seems like nothing's different. Then, after enough miles, the car is in a completely different place, a totally different course. This is the way to lasting change, to guaranteed metamorphosis. When someone wants a major turn-around in their health, for example, I always recommend making one small change a day. In a year, they'll have made 365 little improvements, which adds up to a big difference. And they'll have made new habits and the stamina to maintain them, encouraged by the changes they notice in their life, how they feel, etc. I encourage treating anything important as a marathon, not a sprint, and digging in for the long haul.

It's true that massive change is overdue: in the way we treat each other, our world, and ourselves. But I don't have the dynamite, nor a flair for drama. Instead, I just make one improvement at a time, stabilize it, and then see where

> "Greater than the tread of mighty armies is *an idea whose time has come*." - Victor Hugo

I'm at. I've gotten excited and gung-ho about a lot of things in my life, but I've noticed that permanent and powerful transformation has come about from a sustained 5% turn of the wheel. If you're different, that's awesome, together I hope we can make something really magical happen.

Everyone but the Kitchen Sink: Modernization, McDonald's, and Hyper-Maturation

I'd like to make it clear that this book is for absolutely everyone. The ways of making and preparing food in here aren't just for already-organic urban yoga hipster families; they're for the low-income families that can't afford fresh vegetables, communities and aid-workers in developing countries, and the one-third of American kids that eat fast food every day.

Evolution is slow; it certainly can't keep up with the modernization of our diets. Our Paleolithic hunter-gatherer ancestors lived on hundreds of different wild plant sources, some meat (in the few climates where killing a creature that was running or fighting for its life was less effort than foraging for edible plants), and thereby guaranteed themselves a vast array of potent, living nutrients. Just to put it in perspective, of the food crops grown in 1900, 97% were extinct in 2000, just a hundred years later. And we're talking about the vast changes in lifestyle over the course of half a million years, while our basic biology has stayed the same. In the prehistoric world, starch, fat, and salt were rare commodities that our brains were programmed to seek out with the fervor of junkies. Now, they are available on every street corner in the developed world, and the fast food "restaurants" that offer them claim different characteristics and even different cultures. Starch, fat, and salt are found in almost every case in the precise proportions that mirror the cravings imprinted in our very genes, with lab-concocted cocktails of smells pumped into the air to lure our Paleolithic minds in the door.

Ten thousand years ago (a time frame too short to cause many genetic changes, though one exception is the continued production of lactase, the milk enzyme, in about 25% of post-nursing humans), our ancestors went from a wild food diet totally free of grains to an agricultural lifestyle, in a move that author and UCLA Professor of Physiology Dr. Jared Diamond calls "The Worst Mistake in the History of the Human Race", in his essay of the same name. Our forefathers began growing not the crops that would protect the delicate balance of their health and longevity, but the ones that were the easiest to cultivate, harvest, and store: wheat, rice, and corn began providing the most calories to humanity. The average lifespan promptly dropped seven years[2].

It's no surprise that we're not cut out for the amount of starch, salt and particularly fat in our diet, as it's quickly killing us; heart disease, diabetes, and cancer are all linked to a diet too high in these foods. McDonalds lost two CEOs in a single year to diet-related diseases (2004): heart attack and colon cancer[3]. The majority of Americans are on at least one prescription drug to treat type-2 diabetes, cholesterol, and high blood pressure, all of which are directly related to starch, fat, or salt.

Less lethal but just as alarming are the effects of diets high in trans- and saturated fats on children. The number of overweight children has tripled in the last three decades. Kids' menus at sit-down restaurants are usually much worse than the adults'. Our schools are "7-11's with books" (Yale diet expert Kelly Brownell). Shortened and less happy lives will be the obvious result, but there are more nefarious effects as well. Throughout most of our species' history, female sexual maturity was reached at 17 ½ to 18 years old. In 1900, the age had dropped to 15 ½ in

---

[2] Pia Bennike, *Paleopathology of Danish Skeletons* [Copenhagen: Almquist and Wiskell, 1985]; and N-G Gejvall, *Westerhu: Medeviel Populations and Church in the Light of Skeletal Remains* [Lund: Hakan Ohlssons Boktryckeri, 1960]

[3] I'd like to add, however, that the second CEO, Australian Charlie Bell, perhaps prompted by the release of the documentary film Super Size Me criticizing the health of McDonald's food, led efforts to add healthier choices to the McDonald's menu and offered parents the option to substitute juice and apple slices for fries and soft drinks for their children. The "Supersize" option was also eliminated.

developed countries, and now the average age that girls reach puberty is 11, while many girls mature sexually at 9 or 10. Many researchers originally believed this accelerating change was due to ingesting the hormones given to milk cows and meat animals to speed *their* maturation and growth, but recent studies show that the single greatest cause is the estrogenic effect of additional fat cells in the girls' bodies. Boys show a much less dramatic change, putting them far out of sync with the girls, with the exception of the most overweight boys whose puberty is actually slowed down by the increased estrogen in their body fat. One result of living out of harmony with our biology.

Cultural awareness of the alarming health problems has been steadily growing over the past decade. Ten years ago the public acknowledged that we were in the throes of a losing battle with obesity and heart disease. Two-thirds of Americans were overweight. Obesity-related illnesses killed a third of a million people every year, crippling millions, and costing our health care system almost a hundred billion dollars annually. Overwhelmingly, people singled out their excess weight as the thing they most disliked about their bodies.

In the past ten years, Americans have made a number of choices about their diet and health. The average American has eaten 50% *more* fast food meals and 5 more pounds of sugar per year. Hospital bills related to obesity have risen to $117 billion, and it's estimated that 8 out of 10 Americans are or will become overweight.

In 2004, the World Health Organization proposed dietary guidelines to reduce fat and sugar consumption. The US delegation, which represents the fattest nation in the world, protested these changes, on behalf of the food industry, as "scientifically unproven". While the WHO guidelines call on governments to reduce the unhealthy food advertising aimed at children and use fiscal incentives to limit the availability of junk food and amount of trans fats in the diet, the US Department of Health and Human Services responded that it would be best to use tactics like "better data and surveillance, and the promotion of sustainable strategies that focus on energy balance," hollow and meaningless expressions with just enough buzzwords to dupe the most foolish into thinking that something was being done.

Former senator Peter Fitzgerald noted that putting the USDA, whose first job it is to sell agricultural products, in charge of our dietary guidelines was like "putting a fox in charge of the hen house". The USDA subsidizes farmers to grow high-calorie, low nutrition crops for $19 billion annually, making white flour, corn syrup, hydrogenated margarine, and white rice cost sometimes less than nothing to produce. It becomes these foods that are the most heavily-advertised and make up the bulk of ingredients of fast food, junk food, and school lunches. And while the current administration is offering small subsidies to farms that convert to organic methods, an initiative spearheaded by Mrs. Obama (who is taking much of the ill-placed heat from farmers losing their hard-won handouts), still not a penny goes towards large-scale vegetable farming. I've gone into such detail in these last few paragraphs to illuminate the fact that the very government agencies we've put in place to protect our health and well-being can't be counted on to do that very thing. It is, once again, up to us to take responsibility for our own health.

But it's difficult to choose fresh food when $5 feeds a busy family at McDonald's. Fast and junk food are designed to maximize the cheapest ingredients, and grocery stores can rarely compete. Add to that the time it takes to shop for and prepare dinner and it becomes a daunting task for haggard parents. But an even less expensive meal, both in money and in medical bills, can be had with a deep breath, a few minutes' forethought, and the application of the methods in this book, in even less time than it takes to round up the kids and drive to the transfat pusher on the corner with a winning goatee and bowtie or cute red pigtails. While the dangers of not making a change in our families' diets could be their own encyclopedia, the benefits of doing so are simple: turning our children into vivacious young people with strong immune systems, increased focus and learning - the kids they were meant to be. It's my fervent desire that the mostly unoriginal ideas presented in these books will spread not only to the families that can most easily implement them, but also to the ones that need them most.

Changing Food Habits - Using the Brain for a Change

I doubt that the previous section is enough to shock people into changing their diets. We all know what to do to be healthier: eat more vegetables and less crap, exercise. It's usually not the why nor the what that holds us up, but the how. Willpower or self-talk alone isn't enough to make lasting changes for most people, and just like the force that drives us to continue eating the ice cream our conscious minds know we've had enough of, the reason is our wiring.

The human brain is "an organ so complex we may never fully understand it", says Colin Blakemore, British neurobiologist. There are 100 billion nerve cells in the brain, with ten thousand times as many connections between them. On average, our brains make one million data transfers every second, for the entirety of our lifetimes. Recent studies have found brain cells previously thought to exist only inside our skulls are actually dispersed throughout our entire bodies, amplifying the previous number by orders of magnitude.

In addition to being the miraculous instrument of human achievement, according to David Linden, a professor of neuroscience at Johns Hopkins University, the brain is a "cobbled-together mess… quirky, inefficient and bizarre ... a weird agglomeration of ad hoc solutions that have accumulated throughout millions of years of evolutionary history," he states in his book, "The Accidental Mind," from Harvard University Press. Interestingly, when new kingdoms of species evolved: reptiles to mammals, lower mammals to humans, the brain didn't actually evolve. The entire reptilian brain stayed almost as is, and a new brain was added on top. That means that we're all carrying around the brains of a flatworm, a snake and a primate right next to our advanced thinking capabilities.

The reptilian area of the brain governs habits and emotions and will always choose the easy route if left to its own, literally subconscious, devices. Specifically, the basal ganglia (BG) is a loosely grouped collection of nerve cells located deep within the reptilian part of each cerebral hemisphere. It's responsible for rage, fear, love, lust, contentment, and automatic behaviors like slamming on the brakes, smashing a vase against a wall in startling anger, or opening the fridge to grab the cheesecake before you even know you're doing it. The pre-frontal cortex (PFC) is the newest addition to the human brain, situated right behind the forehead and is in charge of the things that make us human: personality and executive functions: goal-setting, understanding consequences, and differentiating between conflicting thoughts to choose (hopefully) the most enlightened course of action. Basically, it's considered to be the conscious conductor in the orchestration of thoughts and actions in accordance with internal goals. The BG pushes for habitual behavior, while the PFC considers whether or not that deed is going to bring us what we want in the long run. An over-simplified example of this is the drug-addicted brain, which tells the owner in increasingly creative ways that more drugs are needed. We know as observers that the best course of action is to re-shape the desires of the BG by stopping the drug use and consequently changing the messages being sent to the PFC, but just like an addict's brain invents evidence to show that more drug use is the best course of action, within the individual an entirely different story is told.

An iguana or python doesn't respond to coaxing, cajoling, or bargaining; it changes its habits based on repetition, pure and simple. The ritualistic nature of this organ leaves no room for complex emotions (my apologies to the shirtless-under-their-leather-vests guys at the beach with their scaly loved ones.) The time it takes to change a habit depends on how ingrained it is. It's a simple formula. When a wagon wheel goes over the same road, in the same way, an ever-deepening rut results. If the wheel happens to find new ground, all it takes is a little push in the same old direction and the wheel teeters then returns to the rut. But push in a new direction everyday and the wheel will in no time make a new groove, soon becoming deeper than the first and the wheel will easily stay into it, propelling the cart effortlessly in a new direction. Absolutely any habit can change from a rut to a groove, given enough pushes. Research states that simple habits take 21 days to break, and while we're dealing with more complicated lifestyle changes, 3 weeks of daily action and at least the beginnings of changes are guaranteed. If it's a worthwhile goal, these incremental encouragements may, like signposts on the proverbial road, be all that's needed to propel you towards lasting change. It all starts with one action, today.

The pleasure mechanism in the human brain is *extremely* flexible. It will attach to whatever is introduced, whether unconsciously, like heroin or Big Macs, or consciously like whole living foods. We can quite literally re-engineer our evolution, rewire our brains. The brain of someone who has made a habit of a simple sprout salad with homemade vinaigrette will release just as much dopamine, the "pleasure chemical", as a steak and potatoes guy will get from his 20-oz ribeye. The satisfaction of improving our health and the self-esteem that results is enough to pull back the veil of denial that results in actions that destroy ourselves, other creatures, and the planet, and we will soon have a network of habits and beliefs that will make it easy for us to make better choices.

I know from personal experience. As I slowly started eating more and more whole, living, simple foods, I was surprised to find myself craving whole, living, simple foods. If you've never jones-ed after raw baby spinach, it is a pretty wonderful feeling. Processed food started looking like wax fruit, (e.g. - not food), and non-organic food had an unmistakably flat and empty taste. When I travel, I try to sprout as much food as possible and I obviously lean towards authentic and clean cuisines, especially in places like Germany where GMOs are outlawed and almost all the food is grown with traditional organic methods. It's not always possible or polite to eat this way, however, and after a month or two of bratwurst, potato salad, and strudel and the impulses coming from my BG have become quite distorted. It takes just a few meals to start affecting unconstructive change, and about 3-4 times as long to re-position positive habits in the BG. I don't know why negative transformation seems to have more pull than the other direction, but when I get back home I'm bolstered by the fact that the challenging choices I face will soon become effortless, and because of the nature of the basal ganglia-pre-frontal cortex connection, dramatic changes in behavior can make it even easier. Humans have the largest PFC of any animal. Let's put it to use for a better life now and a brighter future for the planet.

Transitioning to a Living Diet

When we're used to cooked food, we usually look for one thing out of our meals, besides the immediate taste sensations: a "feeling of fullness". Living foods nourish our bodies in a completely different, and much more thorough way. This became clear to me during a recent dinner I prepared for some friends and family where one person refused to eat the meal, worrying that they were sure they "wouldn't get filled up from it". That relation grabbed a sandwich from a nearby convenience store and scarfed the fistful of spongy white bread and deli meats while the rest of us enjoyed a living meal. Afterwards, I noticed the general ebullience of the family and the heavy, lethargic quality of that individual. Granted, their food choice may have been healthier if they hadn't had to scrounge for dinner after being ambushed by an alfalfa-wielding hippie, but it's an interesting dichotomy. The "fill your belly", "stick to your ribs" mentality is quite the opposite of being fed on a cellular level, really nourished down to the nerve, where the energy that used to go into digestion and assimilation are already in the food and don't need to be stolen from the body's other processes. It's a different kind of satisfaction with living food when you're used to heavy meats and caramelized starches, but in time you will adjust, if you choose to go that route.

Table 2: Seed/Nut Digestibility Chart

How	What	Why
Toasted	Starches (usually the main component) are caramelized and impossible to utilize. Most vitamins and minerals diminished or gone. Enzymes gone. Some oils are toxic.	Enzymes are destroyed over 108 degrees; most nutrients are destroyed at high temperatures. Heating some oils past 170 degrees creates free radicals and other toxins.1
Raw, right outta the bag	The most difficult to digest and assimilate; heating does destroy (denature the molecular bonds and render inert) some EI's.	Nutrients are in a dormant state and bound with EI's; these rob the body of its own enzymes and more effort than necessary is put into digestion, while less energy than possible is gotten out in nutrition. The living enzymes of the seed are dormant and unusable.
Soaked in water	Easier to handle, but not at peak nutrition.	Soaking starts the germination process, breaking down the EI's so they can be rinsed

		away, but enzymes aren't fully activated, nor are nutrient levels substantially increased, but you're on the right track...
Fermented (in probiotic water, miso, or seed cheese, for example)	Partial probiotic pre-digestion makes protein, healthy fats, vitamins, minerals, and starches present in dormant seed more available.	Beneficial microorganisms go to work on the starches and long-chain proteins, turning them into more easily-digestible simple sugars and amino acids, and thereby taking some of the strain off of the human. Blending with probiotic water releases EI's which are removed by bacteria.
Sprouted	Nutrient levels are at their peak, enzymes fully active. Provides the body with the building blocks of health and an abundance of energy with	

	which to use them.	
Sprouted and Fermented	Bacteria make immunity-supporting compounds you can't get anywhere else. Peak nutrition and complex components broken down into easily-assimilable forms. The benefits of the seed's inherent nutrition and life force, the short-term benevolent action of friendly bacteria on the seed and the long-term advantages to the digestive system as probiotics settle in and prepare to convert everything that comes their way into a greater you.	Plus it tastes freaking awesome.

The "How?"

Sprouting

This is the simplest section of the book, and possibly the most important, because it's the easiest to get started doing and might have the most dramatic effect on your health. There are no microbial cultures to lure into your home with sweets, no artificial lighting to buy, nothing to build, plug in, or even measure, but the benefits of following these simple and straight-forward directions are many. "Sprouting" just means: getting a seed, nut, or grain wet, and keeping it wet, until it grows into a tiny plant. No farm needed, no garden, no dirt. Just some water and something to hold it in – that's it. But the benefits of sprouting are pretty monumental…

- Dramatically improved digestibility - *gives* energy to digestion instead of *taking* it away like most foods.
- Increased nutrition - vital nutrients increase, sometimes thousands of times.
- More food - the mass of the already inexpensive seed you're sprouting increases by a few to a few thousand times.
- Unlocks a world of fresh and vivid flavor, and all of this is available in the dead of winter, while travelling or anytime, with just a couple of days' to a weeks' notice.

…all for about 60 seconds of work a day. Sound worth it?

Hit the Ground Sprouting

Sunflowers are most definitely my favorite sprout, so let's start with those. They can be sprouted in less than a day with just a minute or two of effort. They're ridiculously nutritious: full of calcium and the co-factors needed to use it, just a quarter cup provides the RDA of skin-nourishing, cancer-fighting vitamin E, they're rich in healthy unsaturated fats and fiber, and are 33% protein (more on pg 132). They blend up smooth and their mellow nutty-flowery flavor makes them great for use in virtually any culinary application, from creamy seed milk and nut butter to soups, salads and dressings, desserts and snacks. I'm actually eating some as I write this, with diced golden delicious apples, coconut butter, cinnamon, vanilla and a little raw honey, though they're great just by themselves. Sunflower seeds with the shell on can also be grown in trays with or without dirt into sunflower "micro-lettuce", which is a delicious salad green.

To sprout sunflower seeds, we're going to soak them and drain them. In a glass, jar, bowl, or gumball machine put some hulled (no shell) sunflower seeds. Then cover the seeds with pure water, leaving a little room for the seeds to expand as they drink. Leave them soaking for about 6-8 hours (overnight is good), then dump them into a colander to drain the water, or use your hand to hold them in the glass while the water pours out, then dump them out onto a kitchen towel. We just want to make sure they're not sitting in water. Let them hang out for another 8 hours and you will notice the pointy end of the seed get pointier. This is the beginning of a root system emanating from the seed, and if you continued to rinse them, it would keep lengthening in a curious quest for nutrients. But we don't need to let it go any further and in fact they will start to get a little bitter after a couple of days' growth, as they enter the teenage stage between seed and plant.

That's it. You have in your paws: sunflower sprouts. In 16 hours the seed fats have converted to essential fatty acids, the enzymes have been activated, the carbohydrates have converted to simple sugars and the proteins to usable amino acids, the vitamin and mineral content has increased substantially, and the life force has increased deliciously. Yes, it is that easy. Bon appétit.

Any seed, grain, or nut can be sprouted (grains and nuts are also seeds), as long as it hasn't been cooked, toasted or sterilized in some way. The life's purpose of each sunflower seed is to grow into a big, beautiful sunflower. Each little peanut has the potential to germinate, mature, and reproduce itself into thousands of other peanuts. When you sprout, you make use of that naturally built-in power. There are four reasons sprouted is better than un-sprouted: nutrition, digestibility, quantity and enzymes – let's go into each of them in a little more detail.

Digestibility

Seeds are naturally protected by enzyme inhibitors, or EIs, which keep them from sprouting on top of the ground, or on your counter, or in a bag at the baseball stadium. I'd love to see some burly, body-painted Yankee fan reach into his bag of peanuts and find the green and tangled mass of a peanut shrub growing from his sack of salty snacks. EIs are what keep seeds in a dormant state, able to withstand the high heat of baking in the sun or sitting in a warehouse for 20 Arizona summers, and still able to grow into a vigorous plant when the opportunity presents itself. They also keep us from digesting the seeds very well, and in fact many nut allergies are exacerbated by the presence of these natural chemicals. So getting rid of EIs is very important and makes seeds much better for us. The good news is that nothing could be easier. It's as simple as soaking the seed for a while in water, which makes it think it's time to let down its guard and germinate, and the water will often become cloudy and bubbly - visual evidence that our food is transforming. After the EIs are soaked away, the seed can sprout freely, and all of its resources go into getting ready to shoot up into the sky. As a result, the nutrients become much more available to us. For example, mung beans, which you may have seen in Chinese food as "bean sprouts", have trace amounts of vitamin C normally, but a couple of days of sprouting and there's at least 600 times more. Just soaking seeds and grains before they're cooked will improve their nutritional value a lot, so if you're going to be cooking beans or quinoa or whatever, soak them overnight, drain the water, then cook them. You'll be pleasantly surprised at how this simple step will improve your food. But soaking is just a small step towards unlocking the full potential of a seed.

The simple process of sprouting will, by making digestion easier and more effective, increase energy, immunity, mental functioning, and well-being. When I say that something is more digestible than something else, I'm talking about two things: 1) that it requires less energy by your digestive system to process, leaving more energy for other things, like growing beautiful hair, detoxification, or choosing a great Halloween costume, and 2) that its nutrients are more plentiful and easier to get at. It's not some magical, "take my word for it" kind of thing, it should be obvious to all by having more energy and feeling lighter and happier immediately after eating, no gas, eliminating better, waking up feeling refreshed, and myriad other benefits in the slightly longer run. Everyone is different, and while it's fun and delicious for everyone to play with making nut cheese and yogurt, some may not be able to digest cashews, for example, any other way than soaking and/or sprouting and/or fermenting them. It's a good idea to eat nuts and seeds as far down the Seed/Nut Digestibility Chart on pages 52-54 as possible, but it takes diff'rent strokes. If you're one of these "stomach of iron" people, you may need to plan ahead a little less than the rest of us, though in the long run it sems to all even out: people that overtax their healthy genes or strong consitituations tend to have more problems in those areas as they age than those those who learn healthy habits earlier in life.

Enzyme Inhibitors

Seeds and nuts contain something called "enzyme inhibitors", or EI's, which prevent them from sprouting somewhere that's not a good place to become a plant, like when a seed drops from a tree onto the surface of a rock. Enzyme inhibitors inhibit our enzymes, too, the things in us that not only break up food and grab its nutrients but also heal cuts, get rid of damaged cells, repair and rebuild skin, bones, and organs. EI's keep your own cleansing and healing power under lock and key. The key is water.

One enzyme inhibitor, phytic acid, binds with B vitamins, calcium, zinc, copper, and iron in the digestive tract and can lead to a deficiency in these nutrients. In the recent past, all grains were soaked and/or fermented to improve their nutrition and digestibility. More recently, store-bought oats had soaking instructions printed on the label, but in an apparent effort to be attractive in a world of ever-decreasing attention spans that vital information was replaced with mazes and facts about leopards, leading to a measurable increase in nutrient deficiencies and its symptoms like bone loss and ADD. See a connection? Or were you thinking about leopards lol?

When nuts and seeds are fermented into cheese or yogurt, bacteria go to work on the starches and long-chain proteins, turning them into more easily-digestible simple sugars and amino acids and thereby taking some of the strain off the human. When they're both sprouted *and* fermented it's like your digestive system is in a hammock in Mexico, simultaneously getting a week's worth of office work done every hour... it just doesn't get any better than that.

Enzymes

These are the catalysts of life, the tiny biochemical machines that make it all happen. From blinking an eye to healing a cut, from growing hair to breaking down food into usable parts, enzymes are the superstars. There are three types of enzymes: food, digestive, and metabolic. The first, food enzymes, is the only one we can take in[4]. We have to make digestive enzymes, mostly in the saliva, stomach, pancreas, and other places in the body. Metabolic enzymes are also produced in the body, and the term applies to a wide range of substances that carry out a variety of functions, like cleansing toxins and rebuilding cells, the two basic functions of life. As we age, our ability to produce metabolic enzymes diminishes, and the elderly are increasingly deficient, leading to both the aging process and the rapid deterioration of health after a certain age.

---

[4] if you don't count eating pig pancreas and gleaning some of their digestive enzymes, which is what most bottled enzymes are.

The good news is that these little critters are interchangeable, so if you have leftover enzymes from your lunch, the surplus will get to work on purifying and rejuvenating your body. The *great* news is that there is an abundance of food enzymes in all raw produce, and especially sprouts. Freshly sprouted seeds, wiggling their little tails and all ready to shoot up into a full-grown plant, have many times more enzymes than are needed to digest them, so eating sprouted seeds, nuts, and grains will not only take the burden of enzyme production *off* of your body, it will also *supply* lots of extra horsepower to re-building your age- or stress-weakened systems, supporting your immunity, and making you happy. Eat a meal full of food enzymes, and your organs need to make less or no digestive enzymes. Free nutrients = happy organs. Extra food enzymes convert to metabolic enzymes; free energy for life = happy you.

Joy, enthusiasm, contentment and deep peace are the default emotions of our physiology. Take away the things keeping us un-centered and happiness is ours, consistently and continually. The *really really* great news is that our bodies are so intelligent, that all we need to give them is the extra enzymes and it knows exactly where to apply that energy for our ultimate long-term well-being. So studying how this particular nutrient is for this or that purpose, this food that's supposed to have this certain effect, these things are important, especially if you're combating a specific symptom or ailment, but it's far more important to supply the stimulating tonic of living enzymes to the body and let ancient cellular wisdom figure out what's best done with it.

Quantity

On top of sprouted seeds being the healthiest food on the planet that can be eaten in quantity, they're also cheap nutrition. A couple of bucks per pound for the highest quality organic heirloom lentil seeds – sprout them and the price per pound goes down to 25 cents. Plant a few of these sprouts, grow them into plants and harvet their seeds, and you have real wealth, all from a few lentils or whatever. The same seeds that might have been cooked and eaten in one bite become "seed factories", and can sustain countless people and is a much more effective means of feeding people. Sprouting is an utterly sustainable system of growing food that will not only save you money, but can also provide under-nourished, impoverished populations with an abundance of fresh, revitalizing nourishment.

Sprouting in a nutshell

Sprouting a seed, nut, or grain just means that we wake it up so that it starts the process that ends in a plant. Whether it's a tree, shrub, bush, or grass doesn't matter, because it's not going to make it that far (sorry). All we care about is the prodigious nutritional force being awoken in the thing while the tiny root or stalk is starting to grow out. Anything that's sprout-able is actually a seed or part of one; it has the ability to grow into the entire plant. So we'll call them seeds from now on, whether they're rightly or wrongly called nuts, like almonds, pistachios, or peanuts (which are actually more closely related to peas, and are the underground-growing fruits of the plant. I'm just sayin'), grains like wheat, rye, or quinoa, or beans like pinto, adzuki, or garbanzos. All of these will sprout in exactly the same way. Some very slight modification in techniques and growing times will bring out the best in the different seeds, but the fundamental process is the same.

Here it is:

The Soak: submerge the seeds in clean water overnight (8 hours or so), and then drain them.

The Twice-A-Day Rinse: keep 'em slightly damp and let air get to them for a day or few.

Then... that's it. Nature has made it easy for us to enjoy this super-fresh, vibrantly living and nutrient-packed food. Now let's look at these steps in a little more detail.

Soaking a seed is the big wake-up call it needs to begin germination. Seeds that are sitting on the ground, or the supermarket shelves, are in a state of dormancy or hibernation. They wouldn't want to start sprouting yet, because their chances of growing into a healthy plant wouldn't be very good. They need to be underground, for starters, and have access to plenty of fresh water and nutrients. So unless they get flooded with water, all their nutrients are going to stay locked up. So while water is the key, the lock is the enzyme inhibitors. The nutritional effects of these biochemical padlocks have been discussed, but now you know the botanical reason these exist, the reason they evolved in the first place. Soaking tricks the seed into thinking it's in the ideal conditions to wake up and come back to life.

Clean, but don't get crazy...

The purity of the water is, as you can imagine, pretty important.   The cleaner the water the more enzyme inhibitors are removed, which you can sometimes see as a brown foam on the surface as they're pulled out of the seed. During the soaking, the seeds also begin to take in water and minerals to fuel the sprouting process, so for seeds with a lot of EIs, changing the water, as needed, will ensure that the future little plants have the best molecular building blocks possible for their healthy growth. There are vastly different opinions on the actual type of water that's best for sprouting, whether distilled, reverse osmosis, filtered, tap, etc, but in classic kitchen sink farmer tradition, the simplest is usually the best.

Using distilled water, that is – water that's been removed from any impurities by turning it into steam, then collecting the pure H_2O, by some accounts is actually too clean. Because nature strives for balance, it may actually pull nutrients *out* of whatever it's in contact with, whether a helpless little sprout, or you. Yes, distilled water will extract minerals from your body, particularly your teeth, like microscopic vacuums. Filtered water like reverse osmosis is best for drinking, but the minerals that filtration removes, that are too concentrated for human bodies, are actually good for plants. It works like this: minerals in the soil (tiny rocks in this case) are drawn up the roots of a plant and utilized for growth, fruiting, seeding, etc. Meanwhile, the plant is converting the minerals into forms that animals and humans can use (called chelating, or organically-binding minerals). These chelated minerals eventually return to the soil, whether through compost, manure, or the bodies of the animals who ate them. Then, soil bacteria digest these organically-bound minerals and break the bonds that make them accessible to us, turning them back into little rocks, when they can again be used by new plants. Pretty cool system. The short answer is: we don't use minerals the same way as plants, so go ahead and

All living matter (on this planet, at least) is based on the element carbon. Most people would assume that the increasing carbon in a growing tree comes from the soil, but in fact in comes from the air – carbon dioxide, or CO_2, is breathed in by the plant, the O_2 is split off and the C, carbon, sticks around to make more tree. Another reason free access to fresh air is important for your sprouts to grow up big and juicy.

use tap water with the chlorine (which kills everything) removed[5].

With the exception of chlorine and its relations, those pesky minerals that your drinking water should be without are generally good for your sprouts. A whole-house chlorine filter is best, filtering your sink water is good, but the cheapest and simplest method is to fill a jar or pot with tap water then let it sit. In about 24 hours, all the chlorine (a gas that's lighter than air) will have "floated" out. The water can then be put into a bottle for future use and another "batch" started. It's much easier to be able to fill soak jars and rinse sprouts from the sink as opposed to a jar or bottle of water, but you do what you have to do. I do my sprouting in the shower, because it's a nice humid area with good air flow and low light, but mostly because I don't have room anywhere else. I have a corner shower caddy that holds my jars and bags, but the key is my hand-held chlorine-filtering shower head. I can easily bring in my

---

[5] More on how to do that in a bit. The first step is to start getting sprouts into you asap. Fine-tuning production and culinary details come after, and maybe go on forever, so don't get stuck in the trap of thinking you need to know everything before you do anything. The seed knows. Just let it do its thing. Start today.

trays of grasses and spray everything twice a day. The most work in this method is finding a place to put everything when I actually take a shower, so I try to keep that to a minimum. Just kidding, but if someone doesn't eat things that putrefy in the body like meat and dairy products, junk food, and white sugar and the diet is full of fresh, cleansing green foods, there's no such thing as body odor, even after a week of manual labor or camping.[6]

Air Supply

Like us, sprouts need to breathe. We both take in nutrients and expel wastes through respiration, so good air circulation is key. It's also important for plants for another reason: unfriendly microorganisms thrive in stagnant conditions. This could be still water in a puddle after a rain, our intestines clogged with slow-moving red meat and dairy, or a jar of wet alfalfa sprouts without proper drainage and air flow. In all of these conditions, tough and resourceful microbes - ones we haven't formed a mutually-beneficial relationship with - will move in and there goes the neighborhood. It's an interesting fact that, almost exclusively, "good", or probiotic bacteria, those that live in our digestive system and benefit us in countless ways (see Kitchen Sink Farming Volume 2: Fermenting), thrive in the

---

[6] Other communities, like mine (Portland, Oregon) use chemicals other than chlorine (chloramine here) for disinfectant, which may not evaporate in the same way as chlorine.

presence of oxygen, or aerobically, and the "bad" bacteria, the disease- and poor digestion-causing ones are weakened or killed by oxygen (anaerobic). Oxygen-loving microorganisms are the ones that ferment our many brews and cultures, and excellent health seems to have been made readily available to us by the universal principals of organic chemistry. The perfection of our relationship with aerobic and anaerobic bacteria (along with the profile of available enzymes in living foods being the exact ones we need to digest them) is one of the clearest signs I know of that there's an intelligence and benevolence behind creation. Anyways, we can avoid the infestation of "bad" bacteria – those that will rot our sprouts - by making sure our plants have adequate air flow and good drainage. We can further help oxygenate our crops with the generous use of hydrogen peroxide – an atom of oxygen loosely carried around by water. More about hydrogen peroxide in Kitchen Sink Farming Volume 2: Fermenting Sprouting Methods.

There are a few different ways to sprout seeds, and if you become a virtuoso you may eventually start using them all, as you find this nut is best sprouted this way, and this grain another. For now, though it doesn't get much easier than the vague description above, the following list goes from cheapest to easiest. In true kitchen sink farmer fashion, I recommend you start at the beginning and go down the list until you're comfortable with the time/money ratio.

Remember, each of these techniques does basically the same thing: soak and germinate the seeds, then rinse them periodically to keep them moist and clean off any toxins that may have come to the surface. They vary in ease and application. For example, if you have lots of places to hang bags and not much counter space, you may gravitate toward the bag method. If you have a huge dish draining area and no other room, the jar method is for you. If you need to produce a ridiculous amount of sprouts for a school, for example, and have only the floor in the corner of a room (and power, and are under-budget from the last tax levies), go automatic.

The Jar Method

Get some half gallon canning jars (mason, ball, or some lovely antique ones with colored glass), with 2-part lids, and some porous material that won't corrode or decompose. My favorite is fiberglass window screen, cut into squares plenty big enough, though panty hose or a piece of coarse natural fabric may work too. Take off the lid, put the screen over top the jar, then screw down just the ring part of the lid. Ya got yerself a sprouter, partner.

There are many free alternatives if you need to save cash, or you're the type to serve a loaf of delicious sprouted bread with the question, "Know how much that cost me? Nuthin'. Sprouted the wheat in my sock, ground it with my boot heel and baked it on the manifold of my truck." If so, I'd be proud to be your guest. However, these big jars are very cheap (around a buck each) and are super convenient for a great many things. In fact, I have about a dozen half gallon and a dozen quart mason jars, and use them for everything: drinking and transporting water (there *are* other options than ocean-polluting, land-fill-clogging, sometimes toxic-BPA-containing, not-really-recycling, plastic water bottles), food and bulk grain storage, fermenting, microwaving water to heat and/or sterilize it, and of course sprouting. The quart sized jars are even cheaper, and are available with normal and wide mouths. The wide mouths are the same size as the half gallon mouths, if you choose these you'll only have one size lid in your kitchen. Plus, you may be able to reach your hand in to clean them or pull stuff out. Very convenient.

Note: If you'll be storing prepared food or dry grains, nuts, or fruit in your canning jars (and why wouldn't you?), I recommend a "Pump N Seal", available online for less than $30. Just as you may have guessed, this device allows you to remove the air from your jar, keeping it fresh for longer. If you've been lucky enough to find fresh grains, flours, and nuts, vacuum-sealing them will help preserve their delicate oils, nutrients and flavors. In fact, most flours purchased from the store, whether organic or not, are already rancid, as grains that are milled no longer have the protection of the bran and germ, and the precious oils and oil-soluble vitamins like A and E are lost. Unfortunately, spoiled flour doesn't smell or taste any different, but has a profound effect on nutrition and digestibility. In fact, this rancidity is a common perpetrator in the indigestibility that then is misdiagnosed as a wheat allergy. Grinding flours at home is the best (and cheapest – surprise!) way to preserve their nutrition and taste.

The Bag Method

A few companies, such as Pure Joy Planet and Sproutman sell drawstring sacks that are great for allowing an abundance of oxygen to your teeming progeny. But mesh produce bags work just as well (except on the tiny seeds like amaranth) and cost about 1/10th as much. They're also convenient for storing onions and garlic, and are helpful when soaking seeds with shells, which like to float. Put them first in the bag, then in a bowl or jar full of water, and weight them down with a clean rock or other heavy thing. Same with making sauerkraut and other fermentations, when you want to keep everything submerged under the protective surface of salt water. They can also be used to strain nut milks or "blender juice"; throw a bunch of veggies in your high-speed blender with some water and pour the resulting sludge into a sprout bag over a bowl or wide-mouthed glass. Squeeze out the liquid and you have a pulp-free juice, and though the left over pulp will be wetter than if you'd used a top-of-the-line juicer, I think it's worth saving $400 on a juicer, the room in my kitchen, and it's *much* easier to clean. Just dump the pulp out, turn the bag inside out, slide a hand in like a mitten and proceed to wash your hands. The pulp, just as if it came from a juicer, can add dietary fiber to recipes or be fantastic compost or worm food (see Kitchen Sink Farming Volume 3: Growing for more on vermiculture, worm farming). Sprout bags can also be used as tea bags, saving about 90%, by buying loose tea instead of bagged and measuring it into the bag. A very handy, space-saving, and durable piece of kitchen equipment.

A resourceful soul can find a yard of nylon or hemp and sew them up themselves. Or, lay out a square of material, put the seeds in the middle, bunch up the edges and secure it with a rubber band. I also don't see what would stop someone from using nylon panty hose. Or just hold your sprouting seeds in your hand, sit in a field for a few days, and *really* connect with the lifecycle. Not really, but free options abound. Whatever you use, the bag shape lets in air from all directions and limits mold growth, a definite advantage over the jar method. They're also a snap to rinse, especially if you have a chlorine-filtering, hand held sink sprayer or shower head. I hang my bags from a shower caddy, and in less than 5 seconds I've sprayed pounds of food in several mesh bags.

The Basket Method

This system is best for sprouting leafy greens, such as alfalfa, clover, broccoli, and onion. The process is scientifically the same, of course, that is: soaking the seeds and then keeping them moist and breathing, but the basket gives the plants' roots something to grab onto, and they grow straight up, looking for light with their gracefully unfurling green leaflets. Because of the open top of a basket, more chlorophyll can develop than if you were to sprout these tiny seeds as a jumbled mass in a bag or jar. The square plastic boxes of sprouts that you find in the grocery store (what most people associate with the term "sprouts") are grown this way, in the boxes.

There is a cheap and an even cheaper method to grow delicious alfalfa, wild-tasting clover, vegetal broccoli and spicy radish. The first is to buy a basket or vertical sprouter, usually around $30 and consisting of a few baskets made of plastic with many tiny holes in the bottom for drainage and footholds for roots, and covers/soaking containers. Put a thin layer of seeds on the bottom of the basket and submerge it in the dish full of water. When they're done soaking, lift the basket out, dump the water, flip the dish over and it's now a drain board for the basket. Gently rinse a couple of times a day, making sure not to dislodge the sprouts and their delicate grasp on the textured surface, and in a few days you'll have tall and slender plants, opening pairs of leaves to the sun. You'll want to keep them covered and out of the light for the first couple of days (the soaking dish inverted on top works), then give them time in the sun or artificial light so they'll develop chlorophyll and turn green.

The cheaper method is to use circular natural-fiber baskets and large bowls. Make sure the baskets have a tight enough weave that your little seeds don't fall through, and are untreated. These baskets won't last as long as plastic ones, but in my local Chinatown they can be had for less than a dollar each. You can also use the bamboo steamer baskets that every kitchen seems to have hiding in the back of a cabinet.

Robo-Sprouting (the Automatic Sprouter), for negligent parents

Automatic sprouters are usually large, expensive appliances that make sprouting slightly easier by doing the rinsing for you. When I first looked into them, I expected to find a tube to hook up to a water source and another to run to a drain so I could turn it on and come back a week later to perfect sprouts, but thus far that important feature seems unavailable. The machine still needs to be drained of the used water and refilled by hand daily, which saves a 30-60 second rinse per day. Worth a couple hundred bucks? Not to me it isn't.

There is one product, however, the Easy Green Automatic Sprouter, which is a fairly simple little machine that both sprays the sprouts and drains into a tube, run wherever you like. It saves having to drain the machine by hand which, in my opinion, justifies not doing the whole thing oneself. They're also pretty cheap at $175 and have room for quite a lot of sprouts - about 2 square feet – and also do wheatgrass, so the price could be justified when you're eating all those sprouts you might not otherwise have time to grow. I got mine on ebay for around $90.

Specialty Sprouts:

The Clay Method

An exceptionally easy, albeit specialty, sprouting method. The (don't get turned off by the name) "mucilages" (flax, chia, psyllium, and some mustard seeds, to list some of my favorites) are by far the lowest-maintenance sprouts, and some of the most rewarding. These seeds are protected by not just a shell (insoluble fiber), but also by a slippery gel when wet (soluble fiber) which keeps them hydrated, nourished, and oxygenated, like the albumen of an egg does a baby chick. This means that if you try to sprout them using a jar or bag you'll end up with a slimey mess, but if you just cover them with water in a bowl, they'll sprout beautifully. Make sure to put in plenty of water, as they soak up 2-4 times their size. Mucilaginous seeds can also be grown into leafy nano-greens with similar ease – sprinkle a layer onto the bottom of a sterilized, unglazed clay saucer (the kind kept under houseplant pots) and cover them with plenty of water. Keep them covered with water over the next week, put them in the sun when leaves develop, and you'll soon have tall green sprouts. Pull them up by the roots if you can (which will have attached quite securely to the clay) to get all the benefits of the fiber and essential fatty acidss. An even easier way to do this is float the tray on top of a bowl filled with water. The porous clay will soak up the water in just the right amount to keep the sprouts hydrated. Neat trick.

Bean-Sprouting

Thick, crunchy bean sprouts are common in Asian cuisines, and require a little pressure to take their distinctive shape. Sprout mung or adzuki beans with the bag method and adding a little twist: between rinsings put the sprouting bag in a colander with a weighed bowl on top of it. A rock or full jar with the lid screwed on will work fine. Keep them in a dark place, and in 3 or 4 days you'll have long, fat sprouts to use in salads with an umeboshi-ginger-wasabi dressing, or soy-sauce marinated eggplant sandwiches.

The Dirt on Grass:

Some sprouts have more to offer when they're given the chance at a longer life cycle. So far we've been taking sprouts from embyo (seeds) to infancy (small sprouts) and sometimes, in the case of leafy green sprouts, early childhood. "Planting" the baby sprouts and letting them grow into teen grasses and micro-lettuces is a whole new world of nutrition, life force, and culinary application, and requires a slightly larger skill-set. In the section on growing grasses, such as wheatgrass and sunflower greens, we'll be spreading sprouted seeds onto a thin layer of soil or a fabric-like growing medium, or sometimes nothing at all, as the roots of some seeds will act as their own support structure. By continuing twice-daily rinsings (now called "watering"), you'll have tray-bound fields of 4-8 inch plants that you'll harvest with a serrated knife and eat with a smile. Wheatgrass juice is one of the healthiest and most cleansing foods on the planet, and a salad made of home-grown sunflower greens, piquant mizuna nano-greens, mustard micro-greens, or baby oak leaf lettuce, is a crisp and delicious treat. A tray of greens is also a portable oxygen factory, a handy thing to have in an urban setting. At bedtime, I carry a flat of wheatgrass to my bed like it's a teddy bear. Tray growing is covered thoroughly in Kitchen Sink Farming Volume 3: Growing.

Check out Apendix A: The Wide World of Sprouts - Sprouting Seeds, p.82-p.161, for detailed information about most seeds appropriate for sprouting. Flip through, pick some that sound familiar or fun and get started!

Grid-Iron Chef – The Moveable Farm

Eating well while travelling is surprisingly easy as the forces of nature are the same everywhere on earth. We can employ the natural laws of germination and sprouting anywhere on the seeds we find, buy, or bring to supplement the local cuisine. In places where food is expensive, sprouting your own meals can be a fantastic way to save some green while feeling a lot better than a $25 crepe would make you feel. Your friends will certainly make fun, but when you leave their exhausted selves in a park while you detour to new sights a few times, they'll magically change their tune and start getting inquisitive about the jumble of green hanging in the hotel or host's bathroom, especially as their money exits their wallets and purses as if it had wings.

If you're staying put in one place for a few days and have an adequate supply of water, sprouting is a no-brainer. Bring a few sprout bags and doubled plastic bags full of your favorite seeds on your trip; then soak your seeds in the sprouting bag in a sink or a bowl and then hang it up over one of those or in the shower. The routine of rinsing sprouts twice a day can be disrupted by the stresses and excitements of travel; I do it when I wake up and go to bed just like at home, as consistently as is convenient. If you're growing sprouts that can develop chlorophyll hang them in a sunny window, if possible, when they're ready to green up. The leafy green clover, radish, and alfalfa are among my favorites to grow when away from home because they increase in size a lot and I have to pack less seeds for the same amount of food. They can be eaten at any stage of sprouting for a week and a half or more, and their extra enzymes help with the digestion of new and unusual foods.

I also rock sunflower seeds, of course, because of their quick turn around, high protein and incredible nutrition, as well as for my daily flax.

> "Travel is fatal to prejudice, bigotry, and narrow-mindedness" – Mark Twain

If you're backpacking, sleeping on trains, or otherwise nomadic, you'll have to put a little more thought into it. Fill sprouting bags with seeds inside a Ziploc gallon bag and fill it with water from bottles or, when necessary, sinks or drinking fountains. Then seal the plastic bag, put it inside of another one in case of a leak, and put the whole thing in with your dirty laundry as a last line of defense against gnarly enzyme-inhibitor water. Long flights are the perfect time to start sprouts, when you're already through security you can start them in the airport bathroom sink while waiting for your plane, then drain and rinse them when you land 6-10 hours later. I like to start with sunflower sprouts because they're quick and full of protein. Then I get a few-day mix of peas, lentils, and some flavoring herb seeds going as well as a leafy mix, both of which I rinse and drain for a week, snacking on them the whole time. A mix of fennel, fenugreek, and cardamom are a great after-restaurant supplement, aiding digestion in a variation of the Indian tradition. As much as I love quinoa, needing to be rinsed more than other sprouts means

> "The world is a book and those who do not travel read only one page." – St. Augustine

that it may not be the best choice for travelling, when clean water might be scarce or expensive.

Even grasses can be enjoyed on the road for those with no problem with glutens: germinate and sprout a combination of kamut, rye, barley, or your favorite grass grains in a sprout bag, and instead of planting them in soil, soak the whole mess for 10-20 minutes, two or three times a day in a bowl filled with fertilizer water, in a kind of manual hydroponic system. Fertilizers are diluted with water anywhere from 100 – 700 times, so a couple of ounces of concentrate can last for months, especially if the water is re-used a few times. As explained in Kitchen Sink Farming Volume 3: Growing, soil has two purposes: to hold roots and supply nutrients (including moisture and oxygen), so as the air-bound roots of your grains matte together, all that's really needed is the nutrients. The grasses will grow up towards the top of the bag as it hangs, but won't be accessible to scissors like when they're grown in a tray. Instead, pull an entire chunk of root, seed, and grass off the mass and blend it with water if you have the capability, or just take bites and chew it up. The sweet-sticky grain will mask the intensely nutritive flavor of the grass. The residual fertilizer, if you're using the recommendation of kelp or ocean-based, is perfectly edible. There will be gluten in wheat seeds, whereas there is none in the grass, so if you're sensitive be aware of that.

With the new climates, water sources, foods, and "experiences" you'll be enjoying on your journeys (I pretty much mean drinking), bringing probiotics along with you is also a good idea. Kefir and kombucha can be blended with berries or citrus and sprouted hemp, sunflower, flax and oats, and dehydrated at 108° in leathers, cookies, bars and wraps, and in their dry state take up very little room in your pack. It's actually quite feasible to carry a month's worth of home-grown friendly bacteria in a quart-size Ziploc. With a little bit of planning you can easily enjoy the best food in the world, wherever in the world you are.

Probiotic water (Kitchen Sink Farming Volume 2: Fermenting) can be made on the go as well, sprouting your grain of choice then fermenting whenever you're stopped. Try fermenting in a nalgene wide-mouthed bottle, using a sprouting bag for a breathable cover. Screw the lid on when you're on the move, and take it off when you stop for the night or several hours. Your fermentation will continue whenever there's oxygen, supplying your immune system with vitality-boosting local wild yeasts, kind of like getting vouched for in the microbial community and enjoying VIP status wherever you go.

Growing for Your Pet

Did you ever notice that dog food sits for months or years on unrefrigerated shelves, and it doesn't go bad? Bacteria, with their incredibly resourceful digestion that can literally utilize cyanide for food, want no part of dry pet food. How well do you think your pets will be able to break it down and extract its nutrition for a vibrant life? And for that matter, how different is it from ancient bagged gas-station snacks covered in an orange powder so virulent it can permanently stain clothes? Any and all of the methods in this book are applicable to your pets as well as yourself. Sprinkle sprouts on your cats' wet food. Make dog biscuits by skipping the sweetener in a raw cookie and drying it until it's hard. Sprouted whole hemp seeds are a super food for your parrot.

I'm toying with dehydrating Kombucha SCOBYs as dog chews ("SCOBY Snacks" – credit my best friend from childhood Buell Davidson), the dogs I've experimented on didn't seem to enjoy the unflavored chews (kind of vinegary. Yes, I chew them, too) but did carry them around for a while. I'm considering

"All animals except for man know that the principal business of life is to enjoy it." – Samuel Butler

marinating in peanut butter or another canine favorite, and supplementing the chew with EFAs like sprouted flax seed.

Appendix A: The Wide World of Sprouts - Sprouting Seeds

The following is an alphabetical list of the sprouting seeds in my kitchen, with a few more that I don't use but am very opinionated about. See if you can pick those out.

The symbol is next to my favorite seeds.

Adzuki

A medium-sized red bean, adzukis are poplar in Asian cuisine, made into everything from thick and crunchy bean sprouts to desserts and ice cream. They're high in protein, calcium, iron, phosphorous, potassium and vitamins A and C. One of the few beans that I recommend for sprouting because of their great flavor, digestibility, and nutrition, one still has to be careful with them because invariably a small percentage of them will not sprout; be careful when you're chewing, as a small percentage of them might stay hard and pebble-like. Add them to an Asian-themed sprout mix like mung grown into thick bean sprouts with mustard and poppy (or any mix that begs for a firm, slightly sweet, bright red constituent).

Method: Jar or Bag

Alfalfa

Alfalfa is the sprout most people think of first because they're abundantly available in grocery stores across the world. There's much fuss made over this little guy in the natural and raw food communities and even its name is suffused with fanfare: al-fal-fa, from the Arabic, meaning "Father of All Foods". It's true that alfalfa is abundantly rich in hard-to-find minerals, probably because its roots can reach 100 feet down through the soil with its ravenous appetite for moisture and nutrients. And because it's a leafy green sprout, it also has an even higher abundance of extra enzymes than most, and because of its mild flavor is extremely versatile in food prep, equally at home in salads, wraps, sandwiches, soups, the juicer and the blender. Personally, I think that there are much more interesting, nutritious and flavorful leafy sprouts out there like clover, radish, daikon, and broccoli, but it might just be my inherent need to stay ahead of the curve.

Alfalfa sprouts come into their full glory in about a week with the basket method, but I usually throw sprouts of this type in bags of salad mixes and let them grow for a few days. I am probably lazier than you, however, and when I put in the small effort to grow armfuls of leafy sprouts *en baskette* my digestion is always happier for it. Because they grow so rapidly, they are voracious for air and generate a higher-than-average amount of heat, so are much happier in a bag than a jar.

Some other leafy green sprouts are pretty spicy – radish, clover, celery – and the addition of alfala can help mellow them out.

Method: Basket (preferred) or Bag

Almonds

See "Nuts", pgs 151-161

Amaranth

Amaranth is a tiny South American seed that grows by the thousands in tight cones on a medium-sized red shrub. Popular with both the ancient Aztecs and the Himalayan cultures, this hearty plant can thrive in weak light, poor soil, arid climates and drought conditions.

15-20% protein, which is more than most meats, amaranth also contains the amino acids lysine and methonine, which are necessary for the assimilation of protein but are rarely found in other grains. Amaranth has more calcium than milk and plentiful magnesium and silicon, cofactors necessary for the digestion of calcium which milk does not have.

Amaranth is a deliciously nutty and malty sprout which takes a day to reach its peak and because of its teeny size is best sprouted in a fine mesh bag. Amaranth doesn't require soaking. If you sprout it with anything else, like for "Aztec Bread" (see "Kitchen Sink Farming Volume 4: Homegrown Living Recipes - What to Do with Your Sprouts and Krauts"), it will sink to the bottom of the mixture and hold a lot of moisture so make sure to shake up the bag after every watering. I don't recommend letting it go longer than 2 days after germination, because it will get especially bitter.

Method: Bag

Black Beans

Beans have a diversified portfolio of starches, and it takes a well-educated digestive system to smoothly cash in on their dividends. More often than not, the body has to spend more resources breaking them down and eliminating them than actually assimilating their nutrients. Sprouting (and fermenting) these difficult foods can make them much easier to deal with. I always recommend sprouting everything possible before they're boiled, steamed, baked, or whatever, but I even more passionately advocate sticking with foods that are easily turned into fuel for a vibrant life, namely, those that are still alive themselves. If a food has to be cooked to make it digestible, that food loses the enzymatic life force that inspired me to want to eat it in the first place.

Anyways, black, or turtle, beans are an oval bean with a black skin, cream-colored flesh, and a sweet flavor. Black beans have long been popular in Mexico, Central and South America, the Caribbean and the southern United States. This is not the same bean (fermented black beans) used in oriental cuisines. When sprouting them, let their tails grow as long as the beans themselves, indicating that they've reached the peak of nutrition and digestibility. Black beans are so beautiful and flavorful that I've used them very sparingly in pilafs and crackers, coarsely grinding them and running cold water over them to remove as much un-broken down starch as possible. Again, if you're going to be cooking black or any other beans, sprouting them will add a lot to their flavor and digestibility, especially if they're coarsely ground and rinsed first.

Method: Bag or Jar

Barley

Similar to wheat, barley must be sprouted in the shell and is best grown into a grass. Barley's slightly bitter flavor comes from a more diverse mineral portfolio than wheat, and as a grass is thought to contain more free-radical scavenging antioxidants than wheatgrass. Interestingly, before World War 2, the massive depletion of the soil because of growing one crop over and over again on the same plot of land (monoculture) required the introduction of chemical fertilizers and pesticides and for the first time, the dietary need for vitamin and mineral supplements. Barley grass was dried in tablet form and sold as a primitive multi-vitamin. Since barley grass doesn't have the sweetness of wheat, kamut or spelt grass, it can be grown with these if you're looking for a more nutritionally varied (or "vintage") green drink. "Insta-Grass".

Barely grass has 11 times the amount of calcium than cow's milk, 6.5 times as much carotene and nearly 5 times the iron content of spinach, close to seven times the vitamin C in oranges, four times the B1 in whole wheat flour, and an abundance of B12. It's very high in organic sodium, which dissolves calcium deposits in the joints and also replenishes the lining of the stomach, aiding digestion. People with arthritis routinely use celery juice because of the organic sodium it contains (28 mg per 100 grams), but barley grass contains almost 30 times more (775 mg per 100 grams). As a whole sprout, barley contains 45% protein, twice as much as wheat. It has 5 times the nutrients in the same amount of protein from meat, and in a much more bio-available format.

Method: Grass (preferred), or Bag or Jar

Buckwheat

A mild and delicate microgreen, buckwheat lettuce must be sprouted in the shell and grown in trays on soil, soilless mix, coconut mats, etc. All greens need a good amount of nitrogen, so if you're not using fresh soil with composted manure make sure you fertilize. Cow manure is the best with a little extra boost of nitrogen; chicken and bat guano is a bit too rich - some earthworm castings can be added to potting soil for a similar effect. Soaking the seeds with a little liquid kelp fertilizer should do the trick.

Originally from China and Tibet, buckwheat is a dark green and broad leafed, tender lettuce whose mild flavor is a delicious addition to a salad. It's also a good way to ease into grass juice; start with half buckwheat and half wheat for a milder juice.

Method: Micro-lettuce for salad or juice

Broccoli

A crucifer sprout like kale, cauliflower, and arugula, broccoli sprouts are leafy greens that taste like the full-grown plant and come with an entertaining story.

In 1992, a team of Johns Hopkins University scientists isolated two powerful cancer-fighting phytochemicals in broccoli, glucoraphanin and sulforaphane, which when chewed would combine to form a super molecule called sulforaphane glucosinolate, or SGS, which was particularly effective at fighting free radicals. A 1997 report followed, stating that SGS is in higher concentrations in 3 to 4 day-old broccoli sprouts, at least 20 times the concentration of full-grown broccoli. This discovery was written about in the *New York Times*, and a global shortage of broccoli seed came as a result of the sudden high demand. Then, a year later, John Hopkins University's hastily erected "Brassica Protection Products, Inc.", filed for and received a patent on the method they used to grow broccoli sprouts (to "...exploit the financial benefits of [their] findings" wrote Dr. Paul Talaby in his application), which, according to the lawyers of the sprout farmers that were then sued for infringement, is the same way everyone sprouts them, and the way they grow in nature. BPP formed a partnership with the hulking and deep-pocketed Sholl Group of Minnetonka, MN, a subsidiary of Green Giant Fresh Inc., and promptly started offering sprout farmers a choice: buy an expensive license, stop growing broccoli, or be sued.

"My complaint," said Greg Lynn, owner of Harmony Farms in Auburn, Washington and one of the defendants in the case, "is that Mother Nature should be the one getting the royalties here, and not some researchers milking the money-rich cancer research cow or some corporate opportunists extorting their way into sprout industry domination." Though broccoli sprouts account for only 5% of his revenues, Lynn planned on spending as much as 50% of his yearly sales to fight the suit.

Because the patents had already been issued, they were to be assumed valid by the court and the defendants must present "clear and convincing evidence" otherwise. In order for them to get a summary judgment, the five growers being sued needed to show an argument so compelling and persuasive that "no reasonable finder of fact could conclude otherwise". The sprouters presented this question to the court: "Can a plant, cultivated and eaten by humans for centuries, be patented merely on the basis of a recent realization that it has always had some recently uncovered, but naturally occurring, benefit?"

In the court brief accompanying his ruling, Judge Nickerson wrote, "The Plaintiffs... do not claim that their patents involve doing anything to alter or modify the natural seeds. They are simply germinated, harvested and eaten." He continued, "In construing the claims at issue here, the Court finds that they describe nothing more than germinating sprouts from certain cruciferous seeds and harvesting those sprouts as a food product... Phrases in the claims such as, 'rich in glucosinolates,' or 'containing high Phase 2 enzyme potential and non-toxic levels of indole glucosinolates and their breakdown products and goitrogenic hydroxybutenyl glucosinolates,' simply describe the inherent properties of certain cruciferous seeds. Plaintiffs attempted ... to argue that the claim language, 'identifying seeds which produce cruciferous sprouts ... containing [the desired properties]' introduces a new 'selection' step that was not a part of the prior art. All this step entails, however, is choosing to do something over another, in this case, choosing to grow broccoli instead of cauliflower sprouts instead of cabbage, cress, mustard or radish sprouts. Any process could be prefaced by a similar 'selection' step. Certainly, that one first chooses to perform a particular process cannot be enough to make the process 'new'. Thus, the Court finds that the patents in suit are invalid by anticipation." BPP appealed the case all the way to the Supreme Court, but the ruling was upheld. Five products containing broccoli sprouts are still sold by BPP in grocery stores, including "BroccoSprouts", which are not organically grown and therefore unequivocally cancer-*causing*, and described on their website as "The only product that guarantees a consistent level of sulphoraphane GS", an obviously misleading representation.

Stand up against corporate greed. Fight cancer. Grow and eat broccoli sprouts (which are also high in vitamins A, C, and E, and minerals calcium, phosphorous and magnesium, the cofactors needed to use calcium which are missing from milk.

Method: Basket (preferred) or Bag

Cabbage

The ancient ancestor of broccoli and cauliflower, most people know cabbage from Eastern European soups and the fermented condiments sauerkraut and kimchi. The sprout's distinctive flavor (a lot like cabbage, actually) may take a bit more of a stretch to include into the diet than alfalfa, but the many health benefits are certainly worth it.

Cabbage is rich in vitamin C and glutamine, an amino acid that has anti-inflammatory properties and speeds muscle recovery. Glucosinates, organic compounds consisting of glucose, amino acids, nitrogen and sulfur, are natural pesticides produced by plants in the brassica family, such as cabbage, mustard, kale, horseradish, broccoli and cauliflower, and while they have only a slightly bitter taste to humans, are intensely caustic to insects (taste like napalm). One might think that an organic pesticide might have negative effects on a non-bug, but in fact quite the opposite is true. Many varieties of these vegetables have been developed to remove this slightly bitter taste, but people that eat these cultivated foods are missing out on the anti-cancer benefits of glucosinates, which are being researched for their apparent carcinogen-blocking qualities. Additionally, cabbage is by far the number one vegetable to ferment, and it also has the most naturally-occurring beneficial bacteria of any vegetable. Co-incidence? I think not. I also speculatively theorize that it's the presence of glucosinates that allow these probiotics to thrive, namely lactobacillus, the family that the most common bottled probiotics, acidophilus and bifidus, are in, and have their own set of anti-cancer, anti-inflammatory, and anti-aging properties. **Cato the Elder,** the famed Roman historian, praised cabbage for its medicinal properties, declaring: "It is the cabbage that surpasses all other vegetables." Some question the universality of this statement (ok, just me), but it's definitely up there.

Cabbage seeds are tiny like alfalfa and clover, but with a slightly lower yield of 1 to 5, and sprout just as easily in a jar, bag, or basket. They taste just like cabbage, only a little milder, and are therefore a great garnish to warm tomato soups, or put them in place of sauerkraut in Rueben sandwiches or stadium-style hot dogs. I have yet to ferment them into sauerkraut sprouts, but one day, when I feel like eating something adorable…

Method: Basket (preferred), Bag, or Jar

Chia

Chia is a small mucilage seed from a desert plant closely related to mint, and is both black and white in color. In pre-Columbian times, chia was an important staple in both the Aztec and Mayan diets, and was the basic survival ration of Aztec warriors. It's been said that one tablespoon of the seeds could sustain a runner or scout for a full 24 hours. Banned by the Spanish government in the 16th century after a millennium of cultivation because of its close ties to the Aztec religion, chia is currently experiencing a cultural renaissance, which I hope is due in some small part to their incredible nutrition and not entirely the result of chia-pets and -presidents.

The highest plant source of Omega-3 EFAs (higher than even flax, but not quite as yummy), chia is rich in fiber (over 25%), has 3 times the antioxidants of blueberries, more calcium than milk, and more iron than spinach. Chia also contains high quantities of phosphorus, magnesium, manganese, copper, molybdenum, niacin, and zinc. The Aztecs used chia medicinally to relieve joint pain and sore skin, and I expect both of our cultures can respect the fact that it's so high in anti-oxidants that it will stay fresh for years longer than most seeds, especially as ours deals with a peak oil crisis. As a mucilage, the gel that forms when put in water helps slow down the breakdown and metabolization of carbohydrates and sugar, so it's the perfect thing to add to dessert to keep blood sugar from spiking. Now that modern society is noticing this mighty little seed again, it's being fed to laying hens to increase the omega-3 in their eggs, and chickens and cattle to increase the nutritive value of their meat. If I had to pick an "Official Seed of Societal Collapse", this would be it.

Method: Long Soak or Clay

Clover

Similar to alfalfa, and becoming as popular, clover sprouts have a bit more kick and texture than boring old alfalfa, and are just as versatile.

Method: Basket (preferred) or Bag

Flax

Flax might be one of the most important sprouts for health, as it contains six essential ingredients that are commonly missing from the modern diet. It is unparalleled as a source of essential fatty acids, both kinds of dietary fiber, anti-oxidant lignans, and is an easily-assimilable complete protein. And of course, enzymes when sprouted. It's also surpassingly easy to sprout and tastes wonderful. Everyone should slowly build up to eating a few tablespoons once or twice every day.

Flax seed is one-third oil and the rest is a combination of fiber, protein and soluble fiber or "mucilage", a gummy, slippery substance that makes jar or bag sprouting impossible. Flax must be sprouted with the long-soak or clay methods, which are actually the easiest ways to sprout; just put some flax seeds in a bowl, cover them with water, and in a day many of them will have broken their brown or golden seed coats and sprouted tiny tails. Flax oil is one of the best sources of the rare but essential fatty acid (EFA) omega-3, necessary for good brain function and higher intelligence, mood elevation, inflammation reduction, proper mental development in children, but most importantly (kidding), beautiful skin and hair. (more on EFAs on pgs 95-98)

The protein in flax seeds is easily digested and contains all the amino acids needed for building and maintaining a strong body. Flax's insoluble fiber comes from the shell and acts like a broom, sweeping the colon of toxic material, impacted waste and dried mucus. Flax fiber is excellent nourishment for friendly bacteria in the intestine, which keep disease-causing organisms in check. Twelve percent of flax seeds is mucilage which makes it a gentle, non-irritating, natural laxative. Flax mucilage is perfect for those who have a sensitive stomach, acting as a buffer for excess stomach acids, soothing ulcers or irritable bowel disorders. Dry flax absorbs 20 times its volume in water and can seriously dehydrate a person and become lodged in the colon; sprouting flaxseeds is the best way to enjoy its host of benefits.

Flax is available in two varieties: brown, which is higher in omega-3s and has a harder shell, and golden, which is softer and has a sweeter and milder flavor. If you don't have a high-speed blender, use the golden seeds, because the brown need to be pretty well pulverized, otherwise they can pass through the digestive system intact.

In low-temp baking, the mucilaginous aspect of flax makes it a great substitute for sticky gluten in sprouted loaves. Lightly sprouted ground flax seeds make a light and creamy, mild flavored bread with a spongy quality which makes living tortillas or elastic Ethiopian Injera bread possible. Add a little or a lot of sprouted Kamut or spelt for a more sticky and dense loaf, which will require several times longer to cook. Include some to the pulp leftover from juicing and dehydrate it to make crackers, or add it to young coconut meat to make flexible, thin wraps more pliable than tortillas and nori.

Method: Long Soak or Clay Method

Essential Fatty Acids

Essential fatty acids, or EFAs, carry a slightly negative charge and spread out as a thin, even layer over surfaces. This makes cell membranes soft, fluid and flexible, allowing nutrients to flow in and wastes out. EFAs produce detectable bioelectrical currents, which make possible the vast number of chemical reactions in the body like nerve, muscle and membrane function. This living current is also a measurable difference between alive and dead tissue, and fact of interest in many fields of study, I would think.

EFAs absorb sunlight and attract oxygen; a plentiful supply of oxygen, carried by blood to our cells is fundamental for vitality, pain relief and healing - EFAs are able to hold onto this oxygen at the cells' boundaries, making a barrier against viruses and bacteria. Beneficial bacteria are great in our digestive systems, which aren't really considered to be inside our bodies, because they're not sterile - we don't want any bacteria crossing into our blood or cells, and because EFAs help prevent that they are vital for our immune systems. Because fats are the second most abundant substance in the body (water is first), high-quality EFAs are also important in countless and varied metabolic reactions in the body like fat burning, nutrient absorption, mental health and growth , making them especially important for children. They can substantially shorten the time required for recovery of fatigued muscles after exercise or physical work. Eczema is a severe allergic inflammation, and through their partnership with oxygen, EFAs scavenge allergens from the blood, decreasing inflammation and bringing suppleness and a youthful appearance to the skin. Modern medicine is discovering more and more that many modern health problems are the result of inflammation, so an anti-inflammatory diet with plenty of EFAs is essential for health, especially as we age.

The absorption of sunlight is a curse, however, when the EFA is outside of the living seed. LNA (Alpha Linolenic Acid, an omega-3 EFA), for example, is about five times more reactive to light than LA (Linoleic Acid, an omega-6 EFA). Light increases LNA's ability to react with oxygen by a thousand times. The unsaturated fatty acids with more cis- bonds, like omega-3s, are extremely sensitive to light and will spoil rapidly when exposed to it. So the special nature of the EFAs that make them essential to life - the absorption of oxygen and transformation of solar energy - causes them to decompose when left exposed to air and light, like when seeds are ground and packaged as in the case of flours.

When EFAs and their highly unsaturated long-chain fatty acid cousins are open to the elements, free radical reactions start to take place. Just one photon of light can start a destructive game of telephone, breaking bonds down the line until it peters out around the 30,000 mark. The incomplete molecules join together forming new and toxic compounds. Nature to the rescue: protection from these free-radical toxins is supplied by the fat-soluble vitamins such as A and E, which trap these light-caused chain reactions before they get out of control (and become denatured themselves). These powerful anti-oxidants are always found in concert with EFAs in whole seeds, the perfect container for what might be the body's most vital nutrients.

At best, the refining, bottling, cooking, shipping and storing of EFAs renders them unusable or non-existent, and they can quite easily become carcinogenic. By far the best way to include these vital nutrients in our diets is to sprout the troika of seeds high in EFAs: hemp, flax, and chia, which will offer them the 3-part protection of the seed's shell, free-radical scavengers, and living tissues. It's also (surprise, surprise) the cheapest way: 3 tablespoons of sprouted flaxseed contain 6 grams of omega-3s, the recommended daily allowance, for about 6 cents, in contrast to the 2 dollar shot of bottled EFAs from companies like Udo's Choice and Barleans. Chia provides even more, and of course, both are whole seeds and therefore supply countless other benefits.

All three kinds of EFAs (omegas 3, 6, and 9) are necessary, but special care must be taken to get enough 3. Omega 6 is quite plentiful, available pretty much wherever fats are sold, and we need very little of omega 9, so unless you're eating one bite of celery a day so you can be a prima ballerina, chances are you're fine. But as important as EFAs are to health, the really important thing is the *ratio* of EFAs to each other. The optimal proportion of the 3 and 6 EFAs is 1 omega-3 to 4 omega-6s, 1:4, but the standard modern diet is more often a ratio of 1 to 20 or more. This imbalance causes the body to make fat-soluble hormones called prostaglandins to deal with the excess 6's, wasting valuable globular proteins and essentially creating toxins out of unusable fats. Adult acne is usually created, or at least exacerbated, by this imbalance. This I know from experience, breaking out like crazy when I (as I slowly discovered) ate foods with an over-abundance of omega-6's, avocados and cashews especially. This is why I try to steer raw food chefs away from these ingredients, which seem to be in just about every dish on raw food menus - more like a crutch than an opportunity to feel amazing and alive. Cashews are in fact not raw, but more importantly have little nutritional benefit and a few major drawbacks, such as the toxins and allergens they contain. One of these, urushiol, is the same irritant found in poison ivy, a relative of cashews.

Whenever you eat anything with an excess of omega-6 EFAs (also called oleic or linoleic acids), like cashews, peanuts, olives and oil, almonds, or avocados, make sure to add some sprouted flax seed (or flax oil in a pinch) to the meal to balance out the fats in a healthier ratio.

Garbanzo

Best known as the basis of hummus, garbanzo beans, also called chick peas or chi chi beans, are actually legumes like peas and lentils. Starchy and fairly hard to digest on their own, sprouting simplifies their complex carbohydrates and turns them into a chewy treat in a salad mix; coarsely grinding and rinsing them will remove even more of the tough-to-digest starches. Sprout them alongside sesame seeds for a ready-to-go hummus – just add garlic and lemon and you've got a party in a jar. Large and light brown, these nutty seeds have more iron than any other legume and are a healthy source of saturated fat. They're also high in calcium, potassium and vitamin A.

Method: Bag or Jar, coarsely ground and rinsed after they've sprouted

Hemp-in' Around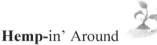

Hemp, the male version of the cannabis plant, has none of the mind-altering chemicals that has made this family of weeds so controversial, and so popular with west coast hip-hop artists. It's unfortunate for the nutritional field, and therefore everyone that eats, that hemp has such a bad… rap? It's an inexpensive and fast-growing source of what may be the best protein found in any food, and certainly best vegetable source of EFAs like omega-3 and -6. Expensive, "essential", and very difficult to find in proper amounts for those that can't or choose not to eat deep-water fish daily because of a growing concern for our ocean's toxicity, ethics, preference, or because they're the 1.4 billion people in the world who live on less than $1 a day. Actually, I find it strange that anyone would want to eat an animal's liver, the organ that is full of fat-encased toxic substances so damaging that the body shut them away instead of risk putting them into the bloodstream to flush away. Fish, especially the ones not from the frigid waters of the arctic (though them too to a lesser degree), live their lives in constant contact with all sorts of toxins, from heavy metals and industrial waste to agricultural run-off and just plain garbage, one patch of which, in the Pacific, is the size of Texas. Plants are the best suppliers of vital EFAs (see pgs 96-99) and lucky for us they're plentiful, cheap, pure, of unsurpassed quality, and quite tasty.

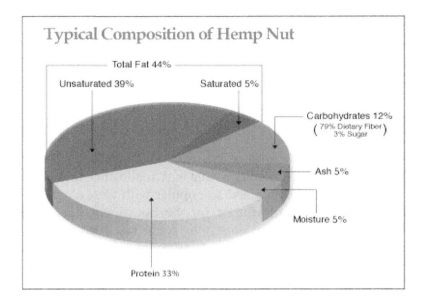

Typical Composition of Hemp Nut

Total Fat 44%

Unsaturated 39%   Saturated 5%

Carbohydrates 12%
(79% Dietary Fiber)
3% Sugar

Ash 5%

Moisture 5%

Protein 33%

Hemp Protein

Hemp protein is the most complete and usable protein in both the vegetable and animal kingdoms. The reason for this is less about the amount than the *type* of protein offered by hemp. Hemp protein, comprising about 35% of its total mass, is a complete protein, containing all 8 essential amino acids needed by the body. It's also about 65% *globular* proteins, **the highest of any food** (this in relation to only about 20% usable protein in beef, and with it a host of problems, like being directly linked to cancer, heart disease, global food shortages and many of the top environmental problems). There are two kinds of proteins: fibrous (or structural) and biologically active (or globular). Fibrous protein builds tissues like muscles, organs, skin, and hooves. Globular proteins make hormones like insulin, hemoglobin and plasma, antibodies in the immune system (also called immunoglobulins – makes sense, huh?), and enzymes, and are therefore responsible for the hundreds of thousands of reactions occurring within each cell at every moment.

Though we can make globular proteins out of any protein we eat, it's much more efficient to take them in in a ready-to-use form. And while conversion of fibrous proteins to usable proteins is an energy-depleting task, globular proteins convert to structural tissue (like big biceps) quite easily as the body's intelligence deciding the best use of each molecule.

These factors make hemp one of the most important foods for overall health and unlike whey, dairy, soy, nut, grain, rice, and egg proteins, it's completely devoid of allergens, making it great for anyone and everyone.

"Plasma, the fluid portion of blood which supplies nutrients to tissue, contains three protein types: serum albumen, serum globulin, and fibrinogen, which together compose about 80% of plasma solids." - Gray's Anatomy, 1978. Hemp protein closely resembles the globulin found in human blood plasma, which is vital to maintaining a healthy immune system.

Hemp Oil

Hemp seed oil comprises 35% of the total seed weight. This oil has the lowest amount of saturated fatty acids at 8% (the ones found in animal products), no trans-fats (the worst ones), and the highest amount of polyunsaturated essential fatty acids at 80% (the good ones) total oil volume. Flax seed oil comes in second at 72% combined total essential fatty acids (though it and chia are higher in omega-3s, the harder to find EFAs). Hemp oil is the only whole food source of both the 'super' polyunsaturated fatty acids gamma-linolenic acid (GLA) and stearidonic acid (SDA), a combination that is required for proper immune system functioning. [7]

"Qualitatively, it is considered desirable to secure amino acids similar to those of human tissues, both as to kinds and relative quantities of the various kinds." - From the "Textbook of Anatomy and Physiology", Kimber, Gray, Stackpole, 1943

---

[7] ("Gamma-linolenic and stearidonic acids are required for basal immunity in Caenorhabditis elegans through their effects on p38 MAP kinase activity" Department of Genetics, Stanford University School of Medicine, Nandakumar M, Tan MW. Epub 2008 Nov 21)

Hemp is also high in:

- Inositol, which promotes hair growth, reduces cholesterol levels, prevents artery hardening, and is calming to the nervous system.
- "Plant hormones", also called phytosterols or phytoestrogens, affect cholesterol absorption, hormone regulation, and cell metabolism.

Potassium, which supports the nervous system and regular heart rhythm and, with the help of sodium, aids in the body's balance of water.

Calcium is essential for a regular heartbeat, strong teeth and bones, and nerve impulses.

Magnesium, a cofactor for calcium, is also needed to transmit the messages throughout the nervous and muscular systems.

Sulfur helps the body resist bacterial invasion and protects it against toxic substances.

Iron facilitates the production of red blood cells and energy.

Zinc is important for a healthy reproductive system and the prostate gland. It speeds tissue regeneration and strengthens the immune system.

- Scientists are studying the use of hemp seed extracts to boost the immune systems of people suffering from immunosuppressive disorders such as AIDS and cancer.

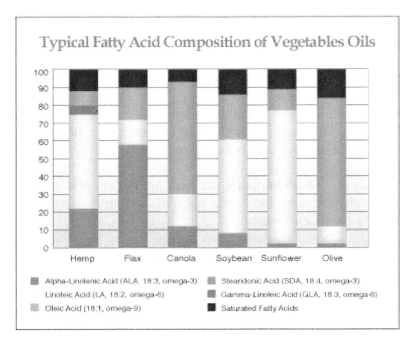

Graph, and previous, reprinted from Gero Leson and Petra Pless',
"Hemp Foods and Oils for Health", 2002

- Edestin is a highly digestible and complete protein
  which comprises about 65% of hemp's total protein.
  This extremely vigorous globulin is so compatible with
  the human digestive system that in 1955 a
  Czechoslovakian Tuberculosis Nutrition Study found
  hemp seed to be the only food that successfully treated
  tuberculosis, a disease in which nutritive processes
  become impaired and the body wastes away. Edestin is
  such a perfect protein that *Science
  Magazine* complained in 1941, "the passage of the
  Marijuana Law of 1937 has placed restrictions on trade
  in hemp seed that, in effect, amounts to prohibition ... It

seems clear that the long and important career of the protein is coming to a close in the US."

Again, the use of hemp seeds has absolutely no correlation with marijuana in the body, and won't cause any adverse reactions in the body or come up on a drug test. Its astounding nutritional profile makes it an extremely important seed that should be a part of everyone's diet. For those in impoverished regions where malnutrition is the norm, the fact that hemp comes from a fast-growing and tenacious plant means that one day its widespread protein-rich nourishment could be possible.

Hemp is only legal today because in the 1930's, when the anti-hemp insanity began in the US, bird seed companies told congress that songbirds would stop singing without this addition to their seed mixes. The compromise was that hemp seeds would be sterilized with infrared heat, making minute cracks in the shell and rendering the seed only semi-viable, even though it's not possible to grow hemp into wacky tobaccy. What this means in the US is that whole organic hemp seeds are available as bird seed and slightly sproutable. The whole seed can be soaked and germinated, then sprouted for a day or two and many of the seeds will start to grow a tiny root. But without the protective integrity of a whole seed, they can start to mold soon after. Stick 'em in the fridge when you see the first tiny tails and enjoy their crunchy benevolence in a myriad of ways.

The seed is also available with the shell removed, called hulled hemp or hemp hearts, and it's automatically sterile. These seeds haven't been heated in any way and therefore all the wonderful oils are still fresh. Though most of the enzyme inhibitors will have been removed with the shell, these seeds also benefit from a two-hour soak. The available enzymes will be activated and in turn the vitamin and mineral content will increase. This is evidenced by the cloudy soak water and change in taste. Until I find a source of organic, unsterilized whole hemp seeds, I use hulled seeds, which I keep in the freezer to preserve the delicate EFAs. Hemp seeds are absolutely delicious, and even if they weren't ridiculously nourishing I would still eat them everyday on their fresh and nutty flavor and creamy texture alone. They're very small, soft, off-white disks, and sprinkled on salads or easily ground into a rich nut butter. Hemp's tastiness makes it easy to enjoy this powerhouse of nutrition and vital life force.

See the "Resources" section for sources of whole and hulled organic hemp seed.

Method:

Whole – Jar or Bag, refrigerate when sprouting begins

Hulled – Soak for 2 hours

Kamut

Kamut is the trademarked name of Khorasan wheat, an amber spring variety with a large, humpbacked kernel. It is an ancient, un-hybridized grain and its high lipid content gives it a buttery taste.

The story goes like this: a US airman in Egypt during World War II was at the bazaar one day when a man who had just finished robbing a pyramid sold him a handful of the 4000-year-old grains he had found there, 36 kernels to be exact, which were apparently the last of their kind. The airman sent the grains to his father, a wheat farmer in Montana, who began to cultivate this venerable and storied grain. County fairs were won, paper boys yelped, and the revival of this near-extinct grain began. Fun story, but unfortunately, at least partially a myth. Most scientists believe Kamut probably survived the years as an obscure grain kept alive by the diversity of crops common to small peasant farmers in Egypt or Asia Minor, and the story was spun by enterprising street vendors, looking to market an inexpensive local grain to wide-eyed US soldiers, one of whom had never before been out of Montana.

Tombs and exotic black market transactions aside, it somehow ended up in the hands of a wheat farmer who planted and harvested a small crop and displayed the grain as a novelty at the local fair in 1964. The legend that the giant grain was taken from an Egyptian tomb was further propagated at this time, and it was called "King Tut's Wheat". In a white flour and new-and-improved crazed America, the novelty of a rich, coarse heirloom grain quickly wore off and it was almost forgotten. Then, in 1977, the one remaining jar of King Tut's Wheat (see a pattern here?) was obtained by T. Mack Quinn, another Montana wheat farmer, who with his son Bob, a plant biochemistry graduate student at UC Davis, spent the next decade cultivating the seeds. The Quinns patented the seed and copyrighted the trade name "Kamut," an ancient Egyptian word for wheat which Egyptologists say comes from the root "Soul of the Earth". Whatever the origin of this special grain and the ethical consequences of patenting seeds, the protection the Quinns have given it has allowed Kamut to keep its heirloom genes unadulterated and it has always been grown organically.

Kamut is higher than wheat in eight out of nine minerals, contains up to 65% more amino acids, the building blocks of protein, and boasts more healthy fats and fatty acids. It's also an excellent source of magnesium, niacin, thiamine, and zinc. But perhaps the most impressive aspect of Kamut is its protein level - up to 40% higher than the national average for wheat. And while its nutritional profile is exciting, perhaps the coolest thing about Kamut is its accessibility to all, including those with wheat sensitivities, gluten allergies, and celiac disease. In a 1991 clinical trial, scientists and physicians tested two different wheat-sensitive populations - people with immediate immune responses and those with delayed responses. In the delayed immune response group, a remarkable 70% showed greater sensitivity to common wheat than Kamut; in the immediate immune response group (the severely allergic) 70% had no, or only minor, reaction to Kamut wheat and were able to continue eating it on a rotational basis. People with allergies should always seek the advice of a trusted health-care practitioner, however, the study concluded that "for most wheat sensitive people, Kamut can be an excellent substitute for common wheat", Elleen Yoder, Ph.D., President of the International Food Allergy Association and head of the team that conducted the study.

Kamut is the best variety of wheat to grow into grass, and alongside spelt, is far better than wheat in food preparation. It gives a rich, buttery flavor to sprouted breads, in contrast with spelt's light, slightly sweet flavor.

Method: Grass (preferred), Bag or Jar for sprouted bread

Lentil

A round, flat seed, like a tiny coin, lentils are commonly found green, yellow, brown and red, though in India over 50 different varieties of lentils are grown. One of the first cultivated plants in human history, lentil seeds have been found in the Egyptian pyramids. The Hunzas of the Himalayas, known for their great physical endurance and long life ("as healthy as a Hunza" is an expression well-loved by many a great-grandparent) ate lentils in abundance. They're said to be one of the most sustaining of all natural foods; during the World Wars, one handful of cooked lentils was the daily ration for many European soldiers.

Soluble fiber increases 300% in 3-4 days in sprouted lentil seeds, which helps lower LDL cholesterol, blood pressure, blood sugar and regulates insulin levels. Fiber of this kind is also a "pre-biotic", feeding beneficial organisms in the digestive tract while simultaneously lubricating the intestines and colon. Lentils are 26% protein and high in calcium, magnesium, sulfur, potassium, phosphorous, and vitamins A, B, C, and E.

Lentils are a member of the pea family but are treated more like beans in food prep, though they're much easier to digest than beans. This gives people interested in maintaining the enzymatic integrity of their foods a hearty and richly-flavored legume to work with that they won't regret later. They sprout easily with the jar or bag method, cook more quickly than beans if you go that route, and give a sweetish, garden-fresh flavor to any dish they're in - brown have the heartiest flavor, green the spiciest, and red are the most mild and lovely to look at.

Method: Bag or Jar

Millet

Prehistoric evidence shows that millet was grown since the stone age in lake regions around Switzerland, and remained popular in Mesopotamia and ancient China. One of the very few alkaline "grains" (actually a seed, which is why it's sproutable and loved by kitchen sink farmers worldwide), millet can help bring our blood pH into balance. Very easy to digest, millet provides both serotonin (a hormone) and tryptophan (an essential amino acid) which are most beneficial when combined. These two nutrients combine to create a powerful team that has several vital functions that effect mood, appetite, sleep, muscle contraction, memory and learning. Millet is also rich in anti-oxidants, magnesium (can help reduce the affects of migraines and heart attacks), niacin (can help lower cholesterol), phosphorus (helps with fat metabolism, tissue repair and energy production) and nutrients that protect against diabetes, cancer and asthma.

Millet must be sprouted in the hull, which isn't how they're usually offered in stores. (See Appendix D, "Resources", pg 173) Hulled, they can be soaked and rinsed before cooking for increased nutrition and

"I don't think most hunger-gatherers farmed until they had to, and when they switched to farming they traded quality for quantity." – Mark Cohen, *Paleopathology at the Origins of Agriculture.*

digestibility, but sprouting them will improve them in countless ways.

Method: Bag or Jar

Alkalinity

Alkalinity is on one end of the pH spectrum, and acidity is on the other. Alkaline foods aren't actually themselves alkaline, but based on their nutritional profile, help bring the body into a more alkaline state. This is the healthy, disease-free state that our nomadic, hunter-gatherer ancestors and animals in the wild enjoy. Acid-forming foods are meat, dairy, alcohol, sugar, saturated fats, and cooked foods, whose starches have caramelized, tissues are lifeless, and nutrients are bound in mostly unusable structures. You knew they were bad for you, now you know (very basically) why. In fact, skeletal records show that the average lifespan dropped by seven years when humans started raising and cooking crops and livestock.[8] Fresh veggies, low-sugar fruits, sprouted seeds, and fermented food and drinks (non-alcoholic, sorry) all contribute to an alkaline system.

The brain, which can't store fat, must get all of its energy from the blood flowing through it. It's hard to extract

---

[8] N-G Gejvall, *Westerhus: Medieval Population and Church in the Light of Skeletal Remains* (Lund: Hakan Ohlssons Boktryckeri, 1960); and Pia Bennike, *Paleopathology of Danish Skeletons* (Copenhagen: Almquist and Wilksell, 1985).

112

energy and nutrients in an acidic environment, which explains why energy and mood drops after the stimulating effects of sugar have worn off. Same goes for cigarettes, caffeine, and cocaine, powerful *alkaloids*, substances that artificially push the blood into an alkaline state. When these compounds lose their potency, the body swings back

into an increased acidity, creating an unhealthy, pendulous imbalance.

Higher acidity in the blood also makes it stickier, not a good thing in a society whose leading cause of death is clogged arteries. When the diet converts to at least 80% alkalizing foods nutrients are more readily absorbed and cellular degeneration (aging) is slowed or reversed. Depression and illness are much less common because of the increase in vitalizing nourishment and energy.

Mung

A smallish bean with a beautiful sea-green color, mung beans are a member of the kidney bean family and are commonly sprouted into "bean sprouts" in Chinese cuisine. Very detoxifying, these beans are high in iron, vitamin C, potassium, and are a complete protein. They are, however, still awfully difficult to digest even when sprouted, and along with adzukis can have some "duds" that don't sprout and feel like a stone in the mouth. The best way to enjoy them, besides saying "mung" to people on the street, is sprouting them fully into thick and crunchy long white vegetables using the pressure method described on page 75 if you'd like to add these fresh, mild legumes to your diet and cuisine.

Method: Bean Sprouts (preferred), Bag or Jar

Oat

Oats are a source of gentle but potent fiber, nutritious, and one of my favorite grains. I was quite surprised when I first concocted a "living oatmeal", expecting to trade my usual light and vibrant feeling for the comforting flavor of a cold-weather breakfast, but found the opposite to be true. Throughout the digestive process my "sproutmeal" gave me a buoyant energy that was a far cry from how I used to feel after eating Quaker Oats. Now this treat is a frequent part of my diet in colder months. See "Kitchen Sink Farming Volume 4: Homegrown Living Recipes - What to Do with Your Sprouts and Krauts" for the recipe.

I may have been previously prejudiced against oats because the many variations of commercially available products remove much of their nutrition and life force. Hulled ground oatmeal is made the same way as white flour and is not much better; steel cut, or groats, are missing many of the key factors that work together with the germ to create complete nutrition and digestibility. Pre-cooked instant or microwaveable products are utterly devoid of benefits. Oats will only sprout in their complete, unshelled form, available as "unhulled" or "sprouting oats" which I've rarely seen in stores, and are very much worth the effort of ordering them online. They are rich in protein, phosphorous (which is essential for the development of the brain and nervous system), and silicon (necessary for the development and renewal of bones and connective tissue). Nutritionally-bankrupt cereal-and-milk or pastries do more harm than good, when "enriched" wheat products with their synthetic vitamins and minerals that are unusable by the body block the cells' recepetors to actual nutrients. Feeding our children living oatmeal for breakfast can help reverse this "overfed, undernourished" epidemic and help make a generation of vibrant young people with full access to their natural intelligence.

Oat is the third leading ceral crop in the US and it fares best in cool, moist climates. This is why oats are such a popular staple in the British Isles of Scotland, Ireland and Wales, and shows that they prefer a dry wit. Today, nearly half of the world's oat crop, more than 4 billion bushels a year, is grown in the United States and Canada. The outer shell of oats is often ground into bran and bottled as a fiber supplement, but it doesn't hold a candle to the effects of whole oat sprout, finely ground in milk, cookies, smoothies, or anything that will merge with its very light, nutty and mildly grassy taste. The first time you try it you may be pleased at the ease of digestion and (especially) elimination. That is to say, a handful of sprouted oats and you'll be B.M.ing like a rockstar. They're also high in vitamins B, E, iron and calcium. The quality and quantity of the protein in oats is far superior to that of wheat and most other grains - oats have twice the protein of wheat or corn flakes. They also contain GLA (the omega-6 essential fatty acid gamma linoleic acid), which helps the body make other EFAs.

Oats sprout very easily, their thick hulls keeping them from retaining water or building up heat, so sprouting them in the jar they soaked in is just fine. Because their hull is so thick, a nice long soak (10-16 hours) is best, weighed down or in a jar filled up and lidded to keep their floaty selves submerged.

Method: Jar

Pea

The crown jewel of the legume family, fresh peas are only available for a month or so in early summer, and I highly recommend taking advantage of them then. They're available frozen during the rest of the year, their nutrients and enzymes in various degrees of degradation. Eating sprouted dried peas is a great way to get their nutrient-rich deliciousness in an easily-digestible form year-round.

Peas have been enjoyed for at least 8000 years for their mild, sweet taste and complex carbohydrates, calcium, magnesium, folic acid, vitamins A, Bs, C, and E. They're also 25% protein. The green variety also have the added benefit of being green, which comes from their natural oxygenating and detoxifying chlorophyll content. A molecule that's only one atom away from our own hemoglobin, which serves our blood's main purpose of carrying oxygen to our cells, chlorophyll is a nutrient that develops in sunshine, and therefore, often a rare commodity for apartment-dwellers.

Easily sproutable with the bag or jar method in their whole form (split peas won't sprout), peas are one of the few sprouts that don't get bitter if they're allowed to grow their roots into long white Fu Manchu beards. They also have a fresh, vegetable-y flavor and I throw them in every salad sprout mixture I make. Peas can also be grown into microgreens in soil or hydroponically. Someone must like them, as they're always available at my local natural foods store in this form, but I find them slightly tough and fibrous, and would rather just make sunflower greens. I also love peas because they're very inexpensive, so it will cost next to nothing to sow a handful of sprouted peas at the base of a houseplant or in a tray, and if you don't like the taste, just leave them alone and soon you'll have a full pea pod factory and your houseplant will enjoy the nitrogen-fixation legumes provide to soil. They're commonly available in green and yellow hues, though a wide range of colors, sizes, and mottling exist. There's even a blue one called the Butterfly Pea that's ground and used as a natural blue food coloring in Thailand.

Peas grow in a uniquely segregated fashion – the root on one side, the shoot on the other, and the spherical pea ball in the middle. For this reason, it's fun to pull them apart while they're eaten, especially for kids.

Method: Jar or Bag

Peanut

More pea than nut, peanuts are actually legumes that, unlike nuts, will poke out a tail when sprouted. Peanuts, or groundnuts as they used to be called by folks dressed like Col. Sanders, originated in South America and are now grown throughout the tropical and warm temperate regions of the world. They were widely cultivated by the natives of the New World at the time of European expansion in the sixteenth century, and were subsequently taken to Europe, Africa, Asia, and the Pacific Islands. Peanuts were unknown in the present southeastern United States until colonial times, where they stayed a specialty garden crop until the civil war, when soldiers on both sides began to grow peanuts for themselves and their livestock. When the war ended, they took their taste for peanuts home. They soon became available from street vendors and at baseball games and circuses.

In 1903, George Washington Carver, an American scientist, botanist, educator, inventor and former slave began researching peanuts at Tuskegee Institute in Alabama. Though peanut butter had been created by then, Carver developed more than 300 other uses for peanuts and improved their horticulture so much that he is considered by many to be the "father of the peanut industry." He recognized the value of peanuts as a cash crop (currently #2 in America) and proposed that peanuts be planted on a rotation basis in the cotton fields where the boll-weevil insect threatened the region's main crop and financial stability. At the time, many people still saw African Americans as intellectually inferior to whites, and the fame of Carver's achievements helped dispel this myth.

Peanuts grow underground, attached to the roots of the shrub. For this reason, they have more enzyme inhibitors than many other seeds, so soaking and sprouting them is non-negotiable to get even a modicum of their nutrition. Peanut butters sold in stores are obviously unsprouted and stale; any vitamins and delicate healthy oils have long since hit the road. To get the most out of them, meals must be at the peak of their freshness and nutrition and prepared right before we eat them. Though it's cheap and easy to do it this way, I haven't seen any products that come close to this integrity that aren't astronomically priced, and on the rare occasions I can find them in big city specialty stores. I'd rather just make them on my kitchen counter or spare bookcase shelf with a handful of humble seeds and couple of minutes' effort.

There are four common varieties of peanut: Virginia, Runner, Valencia, and Spanish; this list goes from largest to smallest. Harder to find, but well worth the search are "wild jungle" peanuts, beautiful heirloom nuts from the Amazon. These peanuts are rich, aromatic and earthy, with a familiar yet exotic flavor and a beautiful mottled red color. As with most wild or closer-to-the-source foods, these peanuts are lower in fat and higher in nutrients. And unlike the hybridized peanuts so many people are allergic to, heirloom peanuts are free of aflatoxin, peanut's allergy-causing component. They do cost 3-4 times more than the others, understandably.

Statistics show that about 1% of adults and 25% of children in the US report an allergy to the peanut, and 25% of these children will grow out of it. (The 1%-6% discrepancy between current and future adults' allergies is probably due to the fact that allergies are more likely to be recognized and reported now than when the adults surveyed were kids.) Recent research in the UK shows that 100% of allergic children were able to build up a tolerance to the allergen through "oral immunotherapy", or taking slightly increasing amounts of peanut flour daily for a 3 week period. It's unclear whether or not this treatment will make peanuts safe for everyone, but it has been shown to protect allergic children from the dangers of accidental consumption of up to ten peanuts, which is in fact the leading cause of food-related deaths.

A pound of peanuts is high in food energy and provides around the same caloric value as 2 pounds of beef, 1½ gallons of milk, or 36 eggs. Cultivated peanuts contain about 30% protein and 45% oil, and are very high in vitamin E (a dietary antioxidant that helps to protect cells from oxidative stress, an inevitable damaging physiological process sometimes referred to as aging), folate (needed for cell division, which means that adequate folate intake is especially important during pregnancy and childhood when tissues are growing rapidly), niacin (a B vitamin that helps to convert food to energy), riboflavin, magnesium, phosphorous, phytochemicals, and fiber.

Peanuts sprout easily in bags and jars, the already-present point growing into a root. They're best after just a day or two, while they retain most of their fat and nuttiness; they'll taste detectibly vegetable after that. Peanuts are dicots like sunflower seeds, meaning that the seed itself is the first leaves the plant will grow into. If you let them grow for a week or more, or plant one in the dirt of a houseplant, point down, they'll grow a few inches then split into a pair of spectacularly large leaves. A fun botanical drama for the young or curious.

Method: Jar or Bag

Quinoa

A staple of the ancient Central and South Americans, quinoa is currently enjoying a surge of popularity. The Incas, who called it the "mother grain", grew quinoa on terraced plots in the Andes Mountains in Peru, Chile, and Bolivia, many of which are still in use today by the descendants of the original farmers. The indigenous people would grind the tiny seeds, which grow in clusters at the end of the stalk of an annual herb, for breads or use them in hearty stews, use the leaves as vegetables, burn the stalk for fuel and even use a sticky resin released from the soaking seeds as soap. But beginning with the Spanish attempt to

120

destroy the Native South Americans culture by burning fields of quinoa and levying severe punishments against anyone caught growing it, and continuing with the mass marketing of refined wheat products, quinoa lost its illustrious status and even developed a negative association among locals, ignorant to their land's potential of being a nutritional mother lode.

Quinoa is 16 to 20% protein, more than any other grain. Even better, it's an unusually complete protein, supplying all the essential amino acids. Not only is quinoa's amino acid profile wonderfully well-balanced, which makes it a good choice for vegetarians and vegans concerned about adequate protein intake, but quinoa is especially well-endowed with the amino acid lysine, which is essential for tissue growth and repair. It has more calcium than milk (the "mother grain") and contains an abundance of the cofactor magnesium, which is necessary to assimilate calcium, as well as silicon, another invaluable nutrient for bone and joint health. It's also very high in iron, B vitamins, phosphorous, vitamin E, and contains no gluten and is therefore not allergy-producing. Its high levels of magnesium relax blood vessels, allowing for increased blood flow and nourishment of the cells and a lower risk of plaque build-up and heart disease. Quinoa can also help prevent type-2 diabetes, as magnesium is also a co-factor for more than 300 enzymes, including ones that regulate glucose and insulin secretion. Quinoa is also a very good source of manganese and copper, two minerals that assist anti-oxidants to combat free radicals that cause aging and cancer.

There are hundreds of varieties of quinoa, from yellow to red, purple to black. The yellow variety is the most common, though an heirloom red variety is starting to show up on supermarket shelves. I prefer this one, which has a more rich and nutty taste, because its ancestors' DNA have been messed with less by selective breeding and chemical influence. All quinoa are naturally coated in a bitter gel called saponin, foreshawdowed above. Before quinoa can be packaged and sold, it must be washed several times to remove this inedible coating, but much of it still remains on the seed. This can be seen in the soak water, which quickly becomes foamy and cloudy. As popular as quinoa is becoming, not many people realize that it must be soaked for 8 or more hours, the water changed at least a couple of times, to remove this digestive inhibitor before it's cooked or sprouted. It also has to be rinsed more thoroughly than the average sprout, because its enzymes inhibitors are more tenacious than most. For this reason, it's best sprouted in bags where a large volume of water can be passed through it easily, instead of filling and dumping a jar many times.

Quinoa is a very quick sprouter, though (24 hours yields a ¼ inch tail, and in a day or two more your crop is at its nutritional apex), so the little bit of extra effort that goes into rinsing is made up in time, and is more than made up for in nutrition and flavor. Quinoa happens to be delicious, with no acquired taste to acquire, which makes it perfect for people transitioning to a less- or no-meat diet. It has a fluffy, creamy,

"About one hundred and fifty years ago, bananas were unknown to the United States and peanuts were only eaten by slaves. So what's to say that an old South American grain called quinoa (pronounced keen-wa) won't become a popular American staple." Author Steve Meyerowitz, Sprouts: the Miracle Food

slightly crunchy texture and a somewhat nutty flavor, is great warm or cold, and mixes well with other grains, vegetables, and flavorings, and is great ground or whole in breads, salads, dips, butters, or sauces.

Method: Bag

Radish and Daikon

A leafy green sprout with a zesty spice, common radish is a crucifer-like cabbage, mustard, and turnip. Its heat is stimulating to the digestive system, helping to remove mucous in the intestines and respiratory system, and fires up elimination. It's both anti-parasitic and antiseptic (good news for Candida sufferers) and supportive to beneficial bacteria. Radish sprouts have 4 times more vitamin A than milk, and more vitamin C than pineapple.

A little bit of radish sprouts go a long way, but they've no equal in meat sandwiches or with other rich foods. Grow them for a week with the basket method or, more efficiently, throw a little bit into a salad mix in a bag or jar.

Method: Basket (preferred) or Bag (for us lazy)

Rice

White rice, like white flour, is made so by removing the bran, or shell. Eliminating most of its nutrients, this process also renders the seed un-sproutable. The milling process that converts brown rice to white also removes about 10% of the product, resulting in an over 40-ton yearly loss of food worldwide. Brown rice will sprout like any other seed, though its sweet, starchy flavor makes it unappetizing raw. Cooked germinated brown rice is far superior to any other form of cooked rice nutritionally because 1) the removal of phytic acid and other enzyme inhibitors that bind nutrients and make them unusable to some degree by the human digestive system (see pg 61 for more on enzyme inhibitors), 2) increased nutrient content, and 3) activated enzymes, which will begin to predigest complex starches and proteins into a simpler and more readily-available form.

Germinated brown rice, or GBR, also tastes much better when cooked than un-germinated rice, and requires less cooking time and therefore retains even more nutrients. Increased 15 times is the amino acid gamma-aminobutyric acid, or GABA, a chief neurotransmitter that helps block anxiety- and stress-related impulses from reaching the motor centers of the brain. A deficiency in this amino acid has been linked to panic attacks and PMS symptoms, and it's used in massive doses as a non-toxic tranquilizer in epileptics. The small amounts available in food can induce calm and serenity, and in its role as a hormone regulator it can increase muscle tone and sexual vitality and promote weight loss. Other remarkable improvements are shown in the amounts of dietary fiber, magnesium, potassium, zinc, E and many B vitamins. It's included in this list of otherwise living foods because rice is so pervasive in so many of the world's cuisines and economies. Rice is the world's main food crop for humans, accounting for more than one-fifth of all calories consumed worldwide[9]. Rice is included in this book to inspire maximization of its potential both as a food and as a commodity.

Incidentally, according to Japanese food economist Ito Shoichi in his 2004 presentation for the Rice Conference held by the Food and Agriculture Organization of the United Nations, there's some evidence that the ancient Japanese germinated all of their brown rice. Another too-common example of modernization changing the inner value of food while keeping the outer form intact. I desperately hope that with the current rapid evolution of both modern science and the popular desire for real food, the best of both worlds will soon be commonplace.

GBR requires a much longer than normal soak time, 1 to 3 days depending on the temperature. The reason rice needs to be soaked so long is its relatively low quantity of phytase, the family of compounds that are activated during germination to neutralize EIs. At 85-100 degrees F, germination takes about 24 hours, at 80 degrees it's about 2 days, and at 60 degrees it's about 3 days (with the soak water changed daily). A low-temperature hot plate or aquarium heater can be used to keep the water the optimal 85-100 degrees. When germination has finished, the rice will change color and the end will begin to bulge. If drained and rinsed for several days, a root system will emerge and the flavor will intensify. Sprouting rice past the germination phase isn't advised, except for specialty

---

[9] Smith, Bruce D. *The Emergence of Agriculture*. Scientific American Library, A Division of HPHLP, New York, 1998

culinary applications like rice pudding and amasake, because it gets pretty sickeningly sweet.

Japanese researchers at the Shimsu University's Department of Bioscience and Biotechnology and the Fancl-Domer Company's Food Science Research Center concluded in 2000, "Continuous intake of GBR can lower blood pressure, improve brain function, and relieve some symptoms of menopause. It also may prevent headaches, relieve constipation, regulate blood sugar, and even prevent Alzheimer's disease and some cancers, including colon cancer and leukemia." As profound as that proclamation is, it's important to remember when reading comparative statements like this that we don't know exactly *what kind* of diet it is being compared to. If you're eating White Castle several times a day, all these benefits and more will most likely apply if you add some GBR. If you're already eating an organic diet rich in living veggies, fruits, and sprouted seeds, you're probably already in good shape. The quotation is included more to give the reader a sense of what the effects of such a simple action like soaking rice before its cooked can have on the undernourished, whether by lack of resources, knowledge, or self-discipline.

When cooking GBR, because the outer shell has been softened by germination, it cooks as quickly as white rice, in a little less than half the regular time.

Method: Long Germination - 1-3 Day Soak, depending on water temperature

Rye

Rye is a relatively young grain; its cultivation began in around 400 B.C, when farmers became interested in a wild grass that grew untamed in the wheat and barley fields in what would become Germany. A hardy plant, rye thrives in poor soil and cold climates, sometimes as far north as the Arctic Circle. In the dark ages, rye was relegated as a food for the poor, and as standards of living improved rye began to take a backseat to wheat. Though it is a "gluten grain", rye has less gluten than wheat, as well as several beneficial properties missing from that "strip-mall of grains". Since it's difficult to separate the germ and bran from the endosperm of rye, it's never been available as a "white" version so its flour retains a large quantity of nutrients, unlike refined wheat flour. Rye contains fluorine, a rare mineral that strengthens teeth and tooth enamel, and its photoestrogenic lignans can help normalize hormone activity. For women going through menopause, this subtle effect can be enough to reduce or prevent symptoms like hot flashes, which are thought to be the result of plummeting estrogen levels.

Because rye has less gluten than wheat, it yields a denser loaf of bread with a rich and hearty, sweet-sour flavor. I recommend a combination of kamut and rye sprouted anywhere you'd use wheat, but it's best grown into its slightly bitter grass form and juiced, which has powerful cleansing properties. You can also sow a little bit into a tray of wheat and barley grasses or use it to make a delicious probiotic water (see Kitchen Sink Farming Volume 2: Fermenting) for a sweet-sour flavor reminiscent of NY delis.

Method: Grass (preferred), Jar or Bag

Sesame

These small, flat seeds are the first recorded seasoning, and have stayed popular for more than 5000 years since. According to Assyrian legend, when the gods met to create the world, they drank wine made from sesame seeds. In ancient India, the seeds were a symbol of immortality, the God Vishnu's consort Maha Sri Devi was associated with sesame seeds, and it's still considered the most auspicious oil next to ghee (clarified butter) in Hindu rituals and prayers. They were used in Ayurvedic medicine to help people achieve a healthy weight, whether they needed to gain or lose. Available in light and dark brown and black, sesame seeds are ground into a nut butter called tahini, a main component in hummus, and are quietly popular in just about every type of cuisine. Especially high in calcium, containing almost 1000 times as much as milk, sesame seeds are also rich in phosphorous, potassium, magnesium, and vitamin A.

Sesame seeds must be in their commonly available shell-on version (which still contains all the healthy oils and fiber) to sprout, though of course soaking the soft, white hulled variety will improve their digestibility, flavor, and nutrition. An easy and quick sprout, soak them for 4-6 hours and sprout them for 2 days. They can be placed on a sunny windowsill for another few hours to develop their chlorophyll as they turn bright green. I love black sesame seeds in my salad mixes and nut butters for their rich and oily middle-eastern taste and gorgeously contrasting color.

Method: Bag or Jar

Soybeans

A complete protein in and of itself, soybeans can produce at least twice as much protein per acre than any other major vegetable or grain crop, ten times more protein per acre than land used for grazing milking cows, and fifteen times more protein per acre than land set aside for meat production. Even so, 98% of soybeans grown in America are used for livestock feed, which yields 20 times less food. Accordingly, Monsanto attacked the soybean first with their bioengineering and legislative muscle; now almost all the soybeans grown in America are from the company's patented "Terminator" seeds that are engineered to only grow once, and genetically-modified to resist the same company's herbicide, Round-Up. This way, farmers need to buy both the especially toxic pesticide as well as new seeds every year instead of using the time-honored tradition of saving their best seeds for the next planting, otherwise the farmer risks government-sanctioned bullying by the company's private police force. This disgusting greed and incredible waste while over 40 million Americans, including 17 million children (one in four) face a daily struggle against hunger.

During the Great Depression, it was discovered that soybeans had the ability to replenish nitrogen in the soil, and great tracts of drought-pummeled dust bowl land were regenerated by this little bean. Henry Ford, of "Built Ford Tough", originally designed the first automobiles and tractors to run on soy oil, with the idea that farmers could grow their own fuel. By 1935, soy was somehow involved in every step of the manufacturing process in his plants, from soy-based paints to plastic panels. He was said to have a suit made entirely of a silky soy fabric, and would give dinner parties with nothing but soybean items on the menu. And you thought I was into this stuff.

An integral part of Asian cooking, soybeans are fermented to make tasty and healthy miso, natto, tempeh, soy sauce, and tamari. The most common usages of soy are in milk and tofu, both of which are unfermented and made from the endosperm, or

> "There's a crack in everything. That's how the light gets in."
> – Ayn Rand, *Anthem*

white part, of the bean and are therefore not much better than white bread. Whole soybeans also contain high levels of lecithin, necessary for the digestion of fat and breakdown of fat deposits in the body. They're also especially rich in iron, omega-3 fatty acids, tryptophan, molybdenum, manganese, fiber, vitamin K, magnesium, copper, B12 and potassium.

Raw soybeans contain "anti-nutrients" that affect humans and animals, and bind and prevent mineral absorption, binding to red blood cells and suppressing regeneration in adults and growth in children, and contain anti-coagulants which keep the blood from clotting. These attributes can be reduced by heat or broken down even more by sprouting, but the only way to enjoy all the benefits of soy with none of the drawbacks is by fermenting your sprouted beans. A few days of sprouting and a few days of fermenting will give you all of the goods and none of the bads. Soybeans can also be fermented into any of the appetizing items listed at the top of the previous paragraph with just a little more effort and patience.

Method: Jar or Bag, and Fermented

Spelt

Spelt is the ancestor of modern wheat, and one of the first known cultivated grains. Perhaps the first grain ever to be used to make bread, it originated in Southeast Asia and was brought to the Middle East more than 9000 years ago. As populations migrated throughout the continent, they brought this hearty and nutritious grain with them to their new lands. Spelt became especially popular in Germany, Switzerland and Austria, where it was called einkorn, or "one seed", for the single grain that grows in each of the plant's small flower spikes. The 13th Century Christian mystic and Benedictine Abbess St. Hildegard said of spelt: "Spelt is the best of grains, warming, lubricating and of high nutritional value. It is better tolerated by the body than any other grain. Spelt provides the consumer with good flesh and good blood and offers a cheerful disposition. It provides a happy mind and a joyful spirit. No matter how it is eaten, spelt is good and easy to digest." Spelt remained popular until the 19th century, and has been making a comeback in the last two decades, from 40 hectares in 1987 to over 3200 in the US just ten years later.

What brought the decline of spelt in the early 1900's is exactly the same reason it's growing in popularity now. Spelt has a tough hull, or husk, that makes it more difficult to process than modern wheat. The husk, separated just before milling not only protects the kernel, but helps retain nutrients and maintain freshness. Also, less pesticides are needed, so even spelt that's not organically grown (which is rare) is less toxic and more environmentally friendly. Wheat dominates the modern world's grains not because of its nutritional content or digestibility, but because of its commercial convenience. It's been bred for centuries to be easier to grow and process, so yields are higher and cheaper, and to have a high gluten content for the production of high-volume commercial baked goods. Spelt does have gluten, but it's water-soluble, making it much easier to digest than wheat, and is therefore an option for some people with wheat and/or gluten sensitivity. And unlike wheat, spelt has retained much of its ancient nutrition and flavor.

Spelt is naturally high in fiber and has up to 25% more protein than wheat. It's plentiful in B-vitamins, as well as mucopolysaccharides, special carbohydrates that are an important factor in blood clotting and stimulating the immune system. Spelt looks generally like wheat or oats, a small light brown cylinder with pinched ends and a deep crease running down the side. Its many health benefits are best enjoyed when it's grown into a highly nutritious grass and juiced, though it can be hit or miss because the necessary removal of the hard shell can sometimes be too much for the seed. It's always fine for sprouting if the inner shell has been broken or much of the germ has been removed, but since grass requires two weeks of growing it can be dicey. Kamut is a more reliable wheat grass; spelt is most useful in sprouted loaves that call for a lighter, sweeter flavor than Kamut's rich butteriness.

Method: Bag or Jar

Sunflower

As mentioned elsewhere, sunflowers are among my very favorite seeds to sprout. In their hulled form they sprout very quickly, less than a day from soak to spoon. They have as much protein as the same weight of chicken breast, and are a rich source of vitamins A, B complex, E, and even D, and minerals including calcium, copper, iron, magnesium, potassium, phosphorus, zinc, and linoleic acid (LA), an omega-6 essential fatty acid. Sunflower sprouts are also a good source of dietary fiber and contain phytosterols, which can help reduce cholesterol levels. They are also abundant in lecithin, necessary for the metabolization of fat and EFAs, both in the diet and stored in the body (lose the love handles).

Sunflower seeds contain the amino acid tryptophan that is responsible for processing serotonin, a neurotransmitter that creates a relaxed and content feeling – for this reason, sunflower seeds combat depression and stress. They blend up smoothly and make a nutty and delicious milk, and add a potent protein boost when used as a base for smoothies, soups, salad dressings, or desserts. And since they're so quickly at their best (8 hours of soaking and 8 hours of sprouting), they can be soaked along with non-sprouting seeds, which will drain as the sunflowers are sprouting. Throw in some pumpkin seeds, walnuts, millet, or hemp hearts, and soak them overnight. Drain them when you get up and let them sprout until you're ready for breakfast, then blend a handful of your mix in water with some vanilla and/or raw honey and/or cardamom, pour the fresh nut milk over the rest of them, add some dried fruit, and enjoy an outrageously easy and nutrient-rich living granola. Save a bit to combine with some honey, drop them on dehydrator sheets and enjoy amazing cookies after dinner.

Shell-on sunflower seeds can be grown into crunchy and succulent microgreens, delicate long white stalks with two thick green leaves on top. They're great added to sandwiches, veggie juices, wraps, dips and soups and can be the main lettuce in a salad. In fact, they may just be the top best-tasting, most nutritious sprouts in both the leafy green and nut-seed sprout categories. This makes them ideal for brand new sprouters and veteran kitchen sink famers alike.

Method: Hulled – Jar or Bag

With Shell: Grown into micro-lettuce

Triticale

A combination of wheat and rye first bred by French botanists as a possible solution to world hunger because it's very quick and easy to grow, and it's rich in simple and complex carbohydrates. It was hybridized in a laboratory setting, and though it's popular as a grass with some folks, I prefer to devote the space on my windowsill to time-tested ancestors of ancient, wild food. Triticale is still under development, though, and is listed here as an option for those working out large-scale solutions to pandemic hunger concerns.

Method: Grass (preferred), Jar or Bag

Wheat

What wheat has going for it is that it's widely available, though in its organic, sproutable form, it's not much more common than its superior cousins, spelt and kamut. It will grow into a nutritious grass and culture the right bacteria for a healthy probiotic water (see Kitchen Sink Farming Volume 2: Fermenting), but the small amount of extra effort to find wheat in its ancestral forms, which haven't been hybridized and genetically manipulated to yield an overly gluey, gummy texture, is well worth it.

For grass growing, it's available as a whole grain, called a berry, in several varieties; you'll want "hard red wheat berries", or one that's specifically labeled for grass.

Method: Grass (preferred), Jar or Bag

Wild Rice

Neither rice nor grain, wild rice is actually the fruit seed of a tall marsh grass native to the Great Lakes region of North America. Harvested by Native Americans for at least 10,000 years, wild rice was collected by canoe in shallow ponds and lakes. Look for organic "heirloom" varieties; descendants of these same plants that yield a shiny, black cylindrical pod with a nutty and satisfying flavor, because much of the wild rice sold today comes from hybridized seeds grown in man-made pools with no circulation for the toxic chemical fertilizers and pesticides that are liberally applied.

Wild rice is rich in calcium, iron, magnesium, phosphorous, vitamins C, E, and B-6, is 15% protein, and is a medium-length sprouter. Its sprouts are best after 4-8 days of rinsing when its hard shell bursts dramatically open to reveal a light-colored, creamy germ center. They're alive and more nutritious just a few hours after they're first drained, so if you're going to cook them, anytime after that is fine. But I recommend you wait and try them when they've opened – they're so soft and flavorful (and full of enzymatic life force) that I bet you'll want to eat them living after all. They are a little on the starchy side, so are best in a salad mix. Their flavor is rich and strong so can add a nice deep nutty taste to an otherwise mild mix. Their unusual color and shape adds a striking contrast to any dish.

Method: Jar or Bag

Herbs and Spices

These seeds will add interesting flavors and/or more subtle, medicinal benefits to sprout mixes; you wouldn't want to eat a handful of coriander or fennel seed sprouts, but throw some in with some pea and lentil sprouts and your pre-dressed mix will have built-in yum. Sprout some garlic seeds for a few days, then add garbanzo and sesame for another day for premixed hummus. I always have a jar of mustard sprouts in the fridge to add to salad dressings, and a tablespoon of cumin sprouts get ground up in anything remotely Latin.

Herbs have a rich history and mystical presence; I'm a fan of foods that are said to both increase vitality by stimulating the healing energy of the body as a whole, and more fancifully, purporting benefits like making one win in court cases (a surprising number of herbs advertise this advantage, actually), and can still be found under a grocery store chain's fluorescent light. Though many herbs are rich in nutrients, I haven't focused on their nutritional profiles here, because the small amount that most people use as a flavoring isn't really enough to nourish on a straight nutrient level. Instead, I'm expounding on their culinary use, fun histories and anecdotes, and their real or perceived effects on health, sometimes in a quite ensorcelled vein.

Herbs have been used since prehistoric times for all manner of denouements, so a good number of their agreed-upon values might just be passed-down superstition. Though there's medical evidence of garlic sprouts lowering cholesterol and fighting off infections and fenugreek seeds have been proven to lower inflammation and lessen dementia, I've always enjoyed herbs more for their culinary uses, leaving their more esoteric properties to my mom's friends that contribute to NPR. However, as a drop of poison in a million gallons of water can have an immediate and potent effect on human health, the subtle energetic qualities of food, the electrons of as-yet unknown chemical compounds vibrating just so, can have equally potent effects on well-being.

As with all seeds for sprouting, it is important to get organic, untreated seeds. Almost all non-organic herbs and spices are irradiated, which renders them biologically (and in all other ways) inactive and unsproutable.

Anise

Anise is a relative of dill, fennel, coriander, cumin and caraway. Many of these relations have been described as having a licorice flavor, but anise is the true taste of licorice - its oils are distilled into the flavoring for licorice candy, and ironically not from the herb licorice. Anise is native to the eastern Mediterranean region and Egypt. It is one of the oldest known plants that's been used for both culinary and medicinal purposes since ancient times; there is evidence that anise was used in Egypt as early as 1500 B.C. To aid digestion, the Romans enjoyed anise-spiced cakes after heavy meals and it was thusly spread throughout Europe by Roman legions. In the Bible, there is mention of paying tithes with anise, and in the 14th Century it was listed by King Edward I as a taxable drug, and merchants bringing it into London had to pay a heavy tax which went towards the repair of the London Bridge. Of the many qualities attributed to anise, I like what one writer puritanically warned: "it stirreth up bodily lust". It was also said to keep away nightmares if placed under one's pillow. Called "Tut-te See-Hau" by Native Americans, meaning "it expels the wind", anise's carminative (or anti-gas) properties have been known since antiquity. It helps with digestion and sweetens the breath, so it is chewed after meals in parts of Europe, the Middle East and India. Anise is a mild expectorant, often being used in cough mixtures and lozenges. It's also antispasmodic (suppresses muscle spasms), soporific (calming, or sleep-inducing in larger quantities) and a few seeds taken with water will often cure hiccups.

Anise is a long and tapered, light brown or greenish seed, about the size and shape of rice. It is a very strong seasoning, so it's best grown as a flavoring agent alongside grains for sprouted breads, and in desserts like fig pudding. Star anise, native to Asia, comes from an entirely different plant. It refers to the dried fruit which will not sprout.

Method: Jar or Bag

Caraway

Caraway seeds are native to North Africa and the Mediterranean, where they're sometimes called "Persian cumin". It's been used for at least 5000 years, making it one of the oldest known spices. Old herbal lore says that caraway can keep things from being stolen or lost, maybe because it was attractive to fowl and was used to keep chickens and pigeons from straying. It was also common for wives to flavor a straying husband's meal with the herb, possibly for the same reason.

It has a sweet warm aroma with a flavor similar to anise seed and fennel. It figures prominently in the cuisines of Germany, Austria, Eastern Europe and Scandinavia, and is traditionally paired with rye, resulting in that robust deli flavor. It's another rice-shaped seed, sometimes striped with lovely alternating bands of green-tinged brown and black.

Method: Jar or Bag

Cardamom

A wild plant native to Southern India, today cardamom is also cultivated in Sri Lanka, Guatemala, Indo-China and Tanzania. Cardamom is the fat seed-pod of a ginger-like plant, ranging in size and color from black and brown to light green, and is best just given a long soak. If you're set on germination, most likely for growing a cardamom plant, the pod's thick coating must be scarified to allow enough water in to the hidden seeds. Shake them in a container with some natural sand, then soak them for 24 hours, rinsing twice daily afterwards. The pod will open and the seeds will begin to sprout in three to six weeks. They can be planted anytime after the first soak, the soil kept warm and tropically moist.

Pungent and aromatic, with a eucalyptusy and lemony perfume, cardamom is said to be a digestive aid and aphrodisiac. It is indispensible in Indian cuisine; try the Mung-Cardamom Sundal in "Kitchen Sink Farming Volume 4: Homegrown Living Recipes - What to Do with Your Sprouts and Krauts".

Method: Long Soak, or scarify and germinate in a Jar

Celery Seed

Though it's relatively unknown in Western medicine, celery seed has been used medicinally for thousands of years in other parts of the world. From ancient times through today, India's Ayurvedic school of medicine uses celery seed to treat colds, flu, water retention, poor digestion, various types of arthritis, and diseases of the liver and spleen. Recent scientific studies have shown celery seed to be effective in the treatment of high blood pressure, cholesterol, and arthritis and can protect the liver from damaging substances such as acetaminophen (Tylenol). It helps reduce muscle spasms, calms the nerves, and reduces inflammation. Oils from the seed also act as a mosquito repellent.

Preliminary studies show that celery seed may help prevent the formation of cancerous tumors in mice[10]. In humans, researchers have found that people who eat a diet rich in lutein, which comes from spinach, broccoli, lettuce, tomatoes, oranges, carrots, and greens, and in which celery seeds are especially high, were significantly less likely to develop colo-rectal cancer.

Celery sprouts can be grown a little or a lot; thrown them into salad mixes or grow them into microgreens to add a

---

[10] Banerjee S, Sharma R, Kale RK, Rao AR. Influence of certain essential oils on carcinogen-metabolizing enzymes and acid-soluble sulfhydryls in mouse liver. *Nutr Cancer*. 1994;21:263-269. Abstract.

beautiful elegance and mild celery flavor to sandwiches, soups, or tuna salad.

Method: Jar or Bag

Coriander

The small round seed from which the cilantro plant grows, coriander probably originated in the Middle East but has been used in Asia for millennium. It's the main ingredient in curry powders, and sprouted coriander makes an exceptional flavoring for salsa, especially for people who don't like cumin.

Coriander has been used to ease stomach upset for thousands of years; in India breastfeeding mothers drink coriander tea to ease their baby's colic. It can alleviate nausea and vomiting. Both the sprouted seeds and full-grown leaves have a cooling effect on the body so it's great for spicy Indian- or Mexican-themed summer meals. Buddhist monks grow coriander in monastery gardens to cool down their sexual urges and help maintain their celibacy.

Method: Jar or Bag, can be soil-grown into Micro-Cilantro

Cumin

Cumin is a medium-sized brownish seed, shaped like a thin tube tapering at each extremity with a tiny stalk attached. It's a stomachic (tones the stomach and stimulates appetite), diuretic (alleviates fluid retention and symptoms of PMS), carminative (anti-gas), stimulant, emmenagogic (promotes healthy menstruation), and antispasmodic (suppresses muscle spasms). Cumin is being researched as a natural way to increase breast size with positive results. In the ancient world cumin symbolized greed; thus the avaricious Roman Emperor, Marcus Aurelius, was given the offensive nickname "Cuminus".

Cumin has a spicy-sweet aroma and a pungent, powerful, sharp and slightly bitter flavor. It's very popular in spicy dishes all over the world: it features in Indian, Asian, Middle Eastern, Mexican, Portuguese and Spanish cookery. Cumin is an ingredient of most Indian curry powders, many Middle Eastern savory spice mixtures, and is the spice most people associate with Mexican salsa.

Method: Jar or Bag

Daikon

Daikon radish is an Asian cousin that's Japan's most common sprout with a thicker stem and slightly hotter flavor. It's otherwise just like a radish, and sprouts the same way (see pg 122).

Method: Basket (preferred) or Bag (for us lazy_____ I mean efficient)

Dill

"Therewith her Veruayne and her Dill, That hindreth Witches of their will." (Michael Drayton's *Nymphidia*, 1627)

Dill is a light brown seed, winged oval in shape with one side flat and the other convex. Appearing in ancient Egyptian writings of 5,000 years ago, dill, from the Norse word "dilla", or "to lull," was once used in sleep tonics to aid insomnia and relieve colicky infants. In the Middle Ages it was used to dispel witchcraft, hence the above quote. Most North Americans associate its aromatic, fresh and slightly sweet flavor with pickles, and in Europe it's a common pastry flavoring. Dill sprouts easily and its pleasant, fresh taste gives a unique flavor to salad mixes, spreads for wraps, and nut cheese.

Method: Jar or Bag

Fennel

A native to Eurasia, this ancient and celebrated member of the carrot family was introduced to North America by Spanish priests, and it still grows wild around their old missions. It has been called the "meeting seed" by the Puritans who would chew it during their long church services. That may have been because of fennel seed's ability to freshen the breath, suppress the appetite (making it a powerful weight-loss agent), or its reputation as an anti-flatulent. The Puritans were a considerate bunch, as long as you weren't a witch. It could have also been for pure enjoyment; fennel seeds have a warm, sweet and aromatic flavor similar to a mild anise.

Fennel is one of my very favorite flavoring herb seeds to throw into a salad mix, as its refreshing licorice-y flavor, which goes with everything always seems to be just the right amount.

Method: Jar or Bag

Fenugreek

Fenugreek, along with just about every other herb seed listed, is a digestive aid. Fenugreek contains natural expectorant properties ideal for treating sinus and lung congestion, reduces

"Money is the most envied and least enjoyed. Health is the least envied and most enjoyed" - Charles Caleb Colton

inflammation, and loosens and removes excess mucus and phlegm. Fenugreek is also an excellent source of selenium, an anti-radiant which helps the body utilize oxygen. But fenugreek's most exciting properties lie in its benefits to diabetics and those with blood sugar imbalances by slowing carbohydrate absorption and inhibiting glucose transport with several compounds, one of which, appropriately called fenugreekine, and is currently being researched for these effects. Fenugreek may also increase the number of insulin receptors in red blood cells and improve glucose utilization, thus demonstrating potential anti-diabetes effects in the pancreas and other organs. The amino acid 4-

hydroxyisoleucine, contained in the seeds, may also directly stimulate insulin secretion. If your blood sugar drops and you get crabby when you don't eat, carry around some fresh or dried fenugreek sprouts and you may notice that everyone around you becomes less irritating.

Fenugreek has a powerful, aromatic and bittersweet flavor, likened by some to burnt sugar. It's used mainly in curries, especially vindaloo and the hot curries of Sri Lanka. It's also a classic component of mango chutney, a key ingredient in Yemenite Jews' unleavened Passover bread, and common in Ethiopian cooking. Fenugreek has mainly been used as a cattle fodder because of its tendency to quickly get bitter, making it a perfect young sprout. Its name actually comes from *foenum-graecum,* or "Greek Hay" in Latin, illustrating this fact. Best for people after only a day or two of sprouting.

Method: Jar or Bag

Garlic Chives

Neither garlic nor chives, this unhurried sprout tastes like a mild cross between the two. Garlic doesn't produce seeds, only bulbs and shoots, so any reference to "garlic seeds" actually refers to this plant. Best sprouted by itself with the basket method, because garlic chives take a week and a half or two to grow into pungent and delicious microgreens, with most of the taste (but much easier on the stomach) than raw garlic bulbs. Garlic chive seeds are also extremely expensive; an actual garlic plant can be easily and cheaply grown by sticking a bulb into a bowlful of soil (see Kitchen Sink Farming Volume 3: Growing) and cutting its fast-growing tubular shoots as needed.

Method: Basket or Grown into Chives in a dish of soil

Milk Thistle

This one is purely for medicinal use – I doubt anyone would eat this hard-shelled, spicy-bitter sprout for its flavor, but everyone *should* for its wonderful liver-cleansing and -strengthening properties. The liver is our second largest organ, after the skin, the first focusing on removing toxins and the second on eliminating them and protecting against new ones. The liver pulls toxic substances from the bloodstream and digestive system, adds co-factors to make them inert, and sends them into the intestines to be eliminated. These toxins can be anything from environmental pollutants, cigarette smoke and smog, to pesticides, free-radicals from heated oils and fried or improperly digested foods, to drugs and alcohol, stress, food allergens, and negative emotions. The Chinese call the liver the "seat of emotions", and many massage therapists will tell you stories of sudden and major emotional releases while working on that area of their clients. But without proper support, the liver fills with poisons and is unable to neutralize them; essentially using the liver's working space for storage.

It's estimated that the average adult's liver is operating at around 20%; at just half-powered liver function it's possible to have radiant skin, limitless energy, ideal weight, and a consistently good mood. You may have noticed that young children in smoking households, who eat fast food for every meal and junk food in between still have glowing skin, boundless energy and enthusiasm. This is because their livers are not yet bulging with toxins and that incredibly powerful and efficient machine is still able to keep up with demand from its punishing bosses. These qualities can be regained at any age with liver cleansing and nutritional and herbal support.

Method: Jar or Bag; sprout for two days and chew them straight like gum if you can take the taste, otherwise toss them in the blender with sweet salad dressings or other blended goodness that will mask the flavor. Sweet cancels bitter and vice versa. They can also be dried, ground, and encapsulated.

Mustard

Though small, spherical mustard seeds are available in a hive of colors (from very light yellow to black); there are two types – normal ("dry") and mucilages. The mucilaginous form of the seed (forms a slippery encasement when wet) is generally of the darker brown varieties and the dry seeds are usually yellow, but there are exceptions to this rule. I prefer the ease with which mucilages sprout – just put them in a dish with some water and you're golden. Actually, different commercially-prepared mustards use different ratios of mucilages to dry, letting them sit for hours or days to achieve just the right dry-to-slime ratio before they're ground up and painted on brats and pretzels.

Mustard is classified in the brassica genus along with cabbage, broccoli, kale, and horseradish, all of which evolved from a common ancestor. This family of plants has a unique root system - after two or three days of sprouting, microscopic hair-like roots will begin to develop when the plant is dry, and will retreat back into the main root after watering. In a few more days, the tiny root-hairs will show up as a distinctive "fuzz" which some people will think is mold but now you know better. They are also quite tenacious and will cling together like puppies in a storm, and have to be separated after a week or so by vigorous rinsing or manual pulling apart. All sprouts produce heat, but mustard becomes especially toasty. For this reason, it's best grown when the weather is less than 80 degrees, and frequent cold-water rinsings can't hurt.

From a study done on the ability of sinigrin, a compound found in black mustard sprout juice, to protect against carcinogenic (cancer-causing) chemicals: "In conclusion, our findings indicate that i) mustard juice is highly protective against B(a)P-induced DNA damage in human derived cells and ii) that induction of detoxifying enzymes may account for its chemoprotective properties. iii) Furthermore, our findings show that the effects of crude juice cannot be explained by its allyl isothiocyanate contents." [11]

In simpler terms, i) black mustard protects the cell against free radical damage ii) if it's in its living state, but iii) they can't figure out why based on isolating its chemical components. I.e. - there's an as-yet unexplainable power

---

[11] *Teratogenesis Carcinog. Mutagen. Suppl. 1:273-282,* 2003 Wiley-Liss, Inc.

in a living seed, a vitality beyond the scope of current scientific knowledge. Hey, they said it, not me.

Mustard sprouts are wonderful in sauces and soups, anything that begs for a bracing bite, and are indispensible in salad dressings not only for their distinctive sharp flavor but also for their role as an emulsifier – a stabilizer that keeps two unlike liquids, like oil and vinegar, from separating.

Methods: Mucilages: (usually brown) Long Soak or Clay

Dry seed: (usually yellow) Jar or Bag, or Soil-Grown into Micro-Mustard Greens

Onion

Like garlic, onion is an allium that takes 2 weeks to sprout, and is ridiculously expensive. Radish is cheaper, quicker, and also adds a bracing kick to dishes. If you love onion, try growing onions or scallions (green onions, the tops can be used in the same way as onions and will continue to grow like grass) in dirt-filled yogurt containers. Your choice: one seed = one continuous 6" plant or 50 seeds = one bite of onion sprouts.

Method: Basket

Poppy

Poppy seeds come in two varieties – "blue" or European, and "white" or Asian. I can't tell the difference in color or flavor, and as far as I can tell the names are based on region, not culinary differences. The opium poppy that's native to the Middle East and also grown in Southeast Asia is a different species. An inert variety grows wild and is also cultivated in Europe and North America. The Eastern variety yields opium and other narcotics, and it is grown solely for this lucrative purpose. Poppy seeds sold for food use (and therefore home sprouts) have none of the alkaloids that comprise any drug. Sorry.

The good news is that store-bought poppy seeds, unlike hemp (which is unnecessarily sterilized, as they can't be grown into an inert relative of marijuana) will sprout beautifully. High in protein and healthy oils, poppy sprouts also make an exotic, metallic-blue colored garnish. Like nuts, they tend to lose a little of their nuttiness and crunch when sprouted, but make up for it with a sublimely subtle sweetness. Poppy seeds are the very smallest seeds in the kitchen sink farmer pantry, so make sure to use a tightly-woven bag or fine mesh screen over your jar. Try them in Strawberry-Poppy Seed Vinaigrette or Almond-Citrus Poppy Sprout Cookies (both in "Kitchen Sink Farming Volume 4: Homegrown Living Recipes - What to Do with Your Sprouts and Krauts").

Method: Bag or Jar with fine mesh

Nuts

For the purposes of this book, nuts are the protein and fat-rich inner section of a hard-shelled seed. Because the shell is removed, nuts don't sprout. They do, however, contain valuable nutrients and their sometimes difficult digestibility and access to their nutrients is greatly improved by soaking. With the exception of wild peanuts, which aren't actually nuts and therefore not in this section (see pg 116) and almonds, which are actually "drupes" (shelled tree-fruit) in heavy rotation in my kitchen and are slightly sproutable due to the protection of their unusually thick inner shell, I don't eat a lot of nuts. Our ancestors probably avoided them in large quantities because of their hard shells; smashing them between rocks to get at the (then) mutilated tiny bite was not a wise transaction of energy, so we never really developed the ability to digest them in quantity. They're not strictly living and are still not a good bargain of digestive effort, especially for those that are used to a 100% living food diet. They can be a great way to transition to less or no meat, satisfying a craving for dense, protein- and fat-rich foods.

Nuts have better than no cholesterol: they're very rich in phytosterols, which block the absorption of unhealthy fats by the cells. These compounds can lower cholesterol and arterial plaque, and reduce the potential of heart disease by up to 15%. [12] There is some evidence, however, that phytoserols can lead to artheriosclerosis, a hardening of the

---

[12] "Consumption of a Functional Oil Rich in Phytosterols and Medium-Chain Triglyceride Oil Improves Plasma Lipid profiles in Men" *Journal of Nutrition* (133): 1815–1820.

arteries, so again nuts are a good transition food but not something that should have a permanently major role in the diet. If they can keep other, worse things out of your mouth then great, and they can be fun to play with in the kitchen, especially for crusts and creamy milk. Of course, their digestibility, fat content, and nutrition is greatly improved by fermenting them into nut cheese and yogurt, as the tenacious chemical bonds that keep them indigestible will be shattered by the work of our little fermenting friends, as the fats and nutrients are the building blocks of healthier compounds in their little paws. See Kitchen Sink Farming Volume 2: Fermenting for more info.

The harder the shell, the more powerful the enzyme inhibitors, so nuts must be dealt with conscientiously if they're to do more good than harm. Soaking them changes their very nature, taking them from hard, dry, and brittle to soft and creamy morsels with complex layers of flavor. They will lose some of their nuttiness, and won't have any of the roasted flavor you might be used to. In fact, soaked green pistachios might be mistaken for fresh peas, and soaked macadamias could be marketed as exotic and delectable fresh fruits. Drained, they'll last a couple of weeks in the fridge, and some of their rich nutty flavor, now more easily assimilable by our digestion, can be returned by low-temp baking or dehydrating.

Because nuts won't sprout, soaking them in salt water will provide all the benefits of soaking as well as enhance the flavor in some cases. The Aztecs soaked their pumpkin and squash seeds in seawater (1 part sea salt to 8 parts water) before they roasted them in the sun, and the process makes quite the delicious snack. Unless they're going to be used for a dessert (and sometimes even then), salt water-soaking makes a tasty, IE-free, vitamin enhanced nut.

Almonds

Today, almonds are grown mostly in California, Italy, and Spain. A law was quietly passed in 2007 which required pasteurization of all California-grown almonds, which presumably kills a pathogen found once on almonds that weren't grown organically and had no immune system of their own, but this heating process also destroys the enzymatic life of the seed. Pasteurized almonds are dead almonds. The only way to buy almonds that are still replete with life is to buy European nuts, the shipping of which can be expensive, or buy unpasteurized almonds directly from the grower at a roadside stand, which a loophole in the law allows. Fortunately, some crafty farmers have set up "internet farmer's markets", where unpasteurized organic almonds and other products can be bought cheaply and with free shipping. Check out the "Resources" section of this book for my favorites.

Almonds are the only alkalizing nuts (see pg 111), and the most nutritious, depending on how you classify them. They are a very complete food, containing generous amounts of protein (12% RDA), healthy fats, and all the "macrominerals", the minerals needed daily in large quantity by the body (except for sodium, which most of us get plenty of already). They contain more than double the amount of calcium in milk, 6 times the magnesium and 40 times the phosphorous, along with a good supply of potassium. They are also rich in many "microminerals", like folic acid, copper and zinc along with 35% of the recommended daily allowance of vitamin E.

They also contain an impressive amount of phytochemicals, a large family of compounds that have been used medicinally for millennia for varied health benefits, and are in use today in modern Western medicine for their effects against heart disease and cancer. Dr. Gary Beecher, Lead Researcher for the in-house research arm of the US Department of Agriculture, analyzed the phytochemical content of almonds and stated: "I have never seen this diversity of phytochemicals in a single food source" in a symposium entitled "Nuts in a Healthful Diet", as a part of the 1998 Experimental Biology annual meeting. Almonds are helpful in fighting heart disease in another way as they contain rhizveritrol, the ingredient in red wine oft-acclaimed at cocktail parties to maintain a healthy cardio-vascular system as an excuse to have another glass. Of course, almonds don't have the drawbacks of alcohol but you will not be popular if you share this fact.

Like most commonly available nuts, almonds have been shelled, but the protective barrier between the hard shell and the soft white flesh of the nut is so thick and fibrous that it will remain intact during the shelling process. This brown skin completely wraps the inner flesh of the nut and is full of enzyme inhibitors, and when fresh, organic almonds are soaked, the water will become quite mucky. Almonds should be soaked for 8-10 hours, becoming deliciously plump in the process. It's best to drain and refill the soak water a few times during the soaking stage, as clean, clear water will bring out the best in the almonds and keep them fresh longer. Because of this relatively thick protective skin, almonds can be sprouted slightly for a day or two after they're drained. Your newly alive almonds should be rinsed once or twice every 8-12 hours, which will cause a small green sprout to form inside the nut, which can be seen if the two halves of the nut are pulled apart and you look closely. Not the dramatic explosion of root and leaf like other sprouting seeds, but we've nonetheless gotten every possible microgram of nutrition out of this special little seed. Because we've removed the almond's natural protection against the elements, they should be refrigerated or low-temperature dried sooner than later, or they will quickly be enjoyed by your local microbial community. As they start to ferment they will get a smell and taste akin to an old-fashioned perfume, which is somewhat delightful in subtle amount but can become overbearing after a few days (kind of like some people who wear old-fashioned perfume).

When sprouted, almonds make a deliciously fresh and nutty butter when ground, and a creamy, frothy white milk when blended with water and strained through a sprouting bag to remove the flecks of brown skin, a totally optional step. The ground skin is slightly bitter and can be used for a skin scrub or dried and used in cookies and breads. This skin is indigestible cellulose, aka insoluble fiber, so if you dry it for future uses don't worry about the temperature or protecting non-existent enzymes and nutrients.

Method: Soak 8-10 hours, sprout in Bag (preferred) or Jar

Brazil Nuts

The seeds of a massive Amazonian tree, Brazil nuts are the largest and oiliest nut in common use, maybe because they have the hardest shell of all time. When soaked, they become quite a bit lighter in flavor as they swell with water. Brazil nuts are great for food preparation as they blend completely and add a subtly exotic deliciousness to a drink or dish. Rich in selenium, a powerful antioxidant for cellular regeneration and protection, Brazil nuts also have sulfur, potassium, and phosphorous.

Soak time: 4-6 hours

Cashews

The seed of a small pear-like fruit that is indigenous to Central and South America, cashews are today primarily grown in India. A relative of poison ivy and sumac, toxins in the shell must be destroyed by cooking the fruit until the nut's outer shell bursts, revealing a light brown hook-shaped nut with a succulent flavor. They have several flaws, unfortunately, such as containing the irritant urushiol, the same toxic oil in poison ivy that causes rashes. Cashews are also extremely high in oleic and monounsaturated fats. These omega-6 and 9 oils are needed in small quantities, but an overabundance will leach the more illusive omega-3's from our system and resulting in a cadre of health problems. For these reasons, I don't recommend over-using them in your food preparation, as most raw food restaurants seem to, with every item on the menu including them. That being said, cashews are pretty much the bacon of the nut world. They make everything taste better, and like bacon bits in salads, foods with cashew pieces in them become a game of "hunt for the nuts". They blend smoothly into a delicious creamy base for soups, sauces, or a whipped dessert topping, which is probably why they're leaned on so heavily by natural food chefs. The heating process destroys any vestigial enzymes that might be present however, and many cashews are treated much worse with the help of radiation and toxic gasses. In any case, they're not a potently enzyme-rich alkalizer like, for example, almonds or sunflower sprouts. Because of the two strikes of an unbalanced ratio of fats and that their life force is cooked away, judicious use is recommended.

Soak for 2-4 hours

Hazelnuts (Filberts)

Grape-sized reddish nuts, hazelnuts have creamy white inner flesh that has an instantly recognizable flavor that's amazing in both sweet and savory dishes. Rich in calcium, potassium, phosphorous, and healthy fats, un-soaked hazelnuts have a slightly bitter flavor. If you already like them, you're in for a real treat when you try them sprouted.

Soak for 8-12 hours

Macadamia Nuts

Native to Australia, the macadamia nut tree was originally brought to Hawaii as an ornamental, with no knowledge of the incredibly delicious nut which would become one of the islands' main cash crops. The sweet and oily marble-sized nut is great in desserts and as a sweet component chopped up in a salad, and their elegant richness makes them a great candidate for cheese (see Kitchen Sink Farming Volume 2: Fermenting).

Soak for 2-4 hours

Peanut

See pg 116

Pecans

An exquisite nut from the hickory family, pecans look somewhat like a walnut (both of which remind me of a dual-lobed wrinkly brain, and traditional medicine draws connections between the nut and the organ) and have a rich, buttery flavor. High in potassium, phosphorous, and vitamin A, pecans are native to North America and grown in temperate southeastern climates. They're thusly marvelous in recipes with an earthy Native American vibe or comforting southern feel, and pecan-crusted or -filled pies are the quintessence of each.

Soak 4-6 hours

Pine Nuts (Piñolas)

Labor-intensively hand-harvested from the inside of certain varieties of pine cones, pine nuts are a torpedo-shaped rich and flavorful addition to tapenade and stuffed vegetables, and are an essential ingredient in pesto (though they are expensive, which is why I make pesto out of walnuts and/or sunflower seeds and sprinkle some pine nuts on top of the finished dish). Extremely high in Vitamins K and E, manganese, copper, zinc and magnesium, pine nuts are also a good source of niacin, thiamine, iron, and potassium.

Soak 2-4 hours

Pistachios

Native to the Middle East, pistachios are a long and lumpy nut with a distinctive green hue. Organic is essential here, as all sorts of nefarious things are done to pistachios conventionally grown, from steaming open the shells before they're ready, to chemically dying the whole thing red to cover up the bruising that happens when they sit on the ground for too long. Natural pistachios are a wonderfully sweet, nutty treat, and should be purchased without the shell if they're to be used for any other reason than keeping my brother and I quiet on road trips in the 1980's. High in protein, copper, manganese, B6, thiamine, and phosphorous.

Soak 8-12 hours

Pumpkin Seeds (Pepitas)

Though not strictly nuts, pumpkin seeds are included in this section because they won't form a root system in the edible form, and will start to rot if they're left moist like sprouting seeds. These seeds of the pumpkin squash are naturally encased in a slippery white shell that's all fiber, both soluble (the natural slipperiness creating a lubricating gel in the digestive tract) and insoluble (the cellulose casing is indigestible and acts like a scouring pad, scrubbing away undigested matter in the intestines and colon). Unlike nuts, this shell doesn't have to be removed from the seed to make it edible, but it does have to be dried before water can soak through it to work its magic on the enzyme inhibitors beneath. That's only if you're harvesting your own pumpkin seeds post Jack-O-Lobotomy; commercial harvesters dry the seed until the shell cracks and is easily removable, leaving the unsproutable flat, dark green seed behind.

Pepitas are one of my favorite nuts for their abundance in healthy oils, vitamins and minerals that are rare in the nut world, high fiber and distinctive taste. They blend up into a creamy froth and contribute equally to all world cuisines, from North and South American to Mediterranean and Asian, maybe because varieties of squash are found all over the world.

More than a third protein, just one cup of pumpkin seeds provides 68% of the RDA, as well as 115% of iron, 185% of magnesium, 96% of copper, 89% of Vitamin K, 162% of phosphorous, and 208% manganese.

*Soak 8-10 hours, this is a good one for salt water-soaking),
1 part sea salt to 8 parts agua*

Walnuts

Like pecans, walnuts are the woody-shell encased fruit from a flowering tree in the hickory family, but are more rich and deliciously bitter than pecans. There are two varieties: the English walnut which is golden brown in color, lightly sweet, and has a higher percentage of the illusive omega-3s than any other nut, and the black walnut which is more intensely flavored and higher in protein, vitamins and minerals. Walnuts are also anti-microbial, especially effective against Candida, and have been shown to decrease inflammation and lower cholesterol, both beneficial to the blood vessels. The hull is used for many medicinal purposes, not least of which is getting rid of parasites in the digestive tract and blood. These benefits are available to lesser degree, but a much better tasting one, in the nut.

Soak 8 hours or so

Appendix B: Sprouting Table

This chart is meant to be a quick and easy reference for sprouting. It won't hurt to do it "right" the first time, so you get it, then do what you like; the general rule is: soak overnight, drain and rinse a couple of times a day until your sprouts are to your liking. Soon you'll be an expert in how to get your favorite seeds, in your climate, to be the best they can be for your particular likes and needs. The seed is the real teacher.

NAME	SPROUTING METHOD	SOAK TIME (HOURS)	SPROUT TIME/DAYS	NURIENTS/PROPERTIES	NOTES
Adzuki	Jar or Bag	Long, 8-10	2	Protein, iron, phosphorous, K, A, C	Adds beautiful red color to mixes; watch out for "duds"
Alfalfa	Basket for Nano Greens; though Jar or Bag is fine if with Salad Mix	Medium, 6-8	2-3 in Salad Mix; 5-7 for Nano Greens	Abundance of enzymes and hard-to-find trace minerals and micronutrients, from its special root system	Very healthy, mild and a little boring. Will grow 16 times their size, so start 1 T seeds for every 1 C. of sprouts desired.
Amaranth	Bag	Zero	0	Protein (including the aminos lysine and methonine), calcium and its cofactors magnesium and silicon	Quick sprouts; will get bitter after 2 days. Though the seeds are small like alfalfa and clover, they'll yield only 30% more sprout than seed.
Black Beans	Jar or Bag	Long, 8-10	1-2	Molybdenum, folate, fiber, tryptophan, manganese, protein, starches	Difficult to digest – best as a garnish, or ground, rinsed, and fermented. Or, if you're going to cook them anyways, it's best to sprout them first.
Barley	Tray Method for Grass; Jar or Bag for Sprouts	Prolonged, 10-12	2-3 for Sprouts; 6-9 for Grass	Chlorophyll, enzymes including SOD, iron, folic acid, C and B-vitamins	Can lower cholesterol and regulate blood sugar. Fairly bitter flavor.
Broccoli	Basket for Nano Greens; though Jar or Bag is fine if with Salad Mix	Medium, 6-8	2-3 in Salad Mix; 5-7 for Nano Green Sprouts; 7-10 for Micro Greens	Cancer-fighting SGS, vitamins A, C, and E, calcium, phosphorous and magnesium	Will grow 16 times their size, so soak 1 T seeds for every 1 C. of sprouts.
Buckwheat	Tray Method for Grass; Jar or Bag for Sprouts	Prolonged, 10-12	2-3 for Sprouts; 6-9 for Grass	Chlorophyll, Iron, Lecithin, Potassium, Vitamins A, and C and Calcium	Mild, very tender leaves are a great addition to a salad or way to ease into drinking grass juice; plant 50% buckwheat to start.
Cabbage	Jar or Bag, never a basket	Long, 8-10	4-8	Very high in vitamin C; glucosinates have anti-cancer and anti inflammatory properties.	One of the most nutritious sprouts. 5 to 1 yield, mild cabbage flavor.

NAME	SPROUTING METHOD	SOAK TIME (HOURS)	SPROUT TIME/DAYS	NURIENTS/PROPERTIES	NOTES
Chia	Long Soak or Clay Method	Continuous Soak	2 days for Long Soak (a small tail may or may not be visible), then refrigerate, 5-6 days for Nano Greens	Very powerful food. The most Omega-3s of any plant source and without the toxic heavy metals of fish sources. Calcium, phosphorous, magnesium, iron, niacin, zinc, manganese, copper, molybdenum	Like flax the world's easiest sprout/ micro green to grow.
Clover	Basket for Nano Greens; Jar or Bag is fine if with Salad Mix	Medium, 6-8	2-3 in Salad Mix; 5-7 for Nano Greens	Vitamins A, B, C, E and K, Calcium, Iron, Magnesium, Phosphorus, Potassium, Zinc, Carotene, Chlorophyll, Aminos, Trace Elements, Protien	Nutrient profile is excellent for women. Will grow 16 times their size, so soak 1 T seeds for every 1 C. of sprouts.
Flax	Long Soak or Clay Method	Continuous Soak	2 days for Long Soak, until the shell opens and a small tail pokes out, then refrigerate. 5-6 days for Nano Greens	Omega-3 EFAs, awesome fiber, complete protein. A recommended daily health boost.	The world's easiest sprout/ micro-green.
Garbanzo	Jar or Bag	Long, 8-10	2-3	Fiber, molybdenum, manganese, folate	Still starchy even after sprouting, a coarse grind and rinse is suggested. Essential in hummus and falafel.
Hemp	Jar or Bag	Prolonged, 8-12	2-3 – refrigerate when tail is as long as the seed; sterilized seeds will stop sprouting and begin to mold after a few days.	Best vegetable source of protein, better than animal by some points of view. EFAs galore, fiber, vitamin E, lecithin, potassium, magnesium, iron, zinc, sulphur, phytosterols, inositol, edestin	Hemp seeds are sterilized by law in the US; they will only grow a tiny tail no matter how long they're grown. Stop after 2-3 days, before they mold.

NAME	SPROUTING METHOD	SOAK TIME (HOURS)	SPROUT TIME/DAYS	NURIENTS/PROPERTIES	NOTES
Kamut	Tray Method for Grass; Jar or Bag for Sprouts	Prolonged, 10-12	2-3 for Sprouts; 6-9 for Grass	40% more protein than wheat, magnesium, niacin, thiamine, and zinc, healthy fats. May be untroublesome to people with wheat and gluten allergies.	Adds a rich buttery taste to sprouted loaves.
Lentil	Jar or Bag	Long, 8-10	2-3	26 % protein and high in calcium, magnesium, sulfur, potassium, phosphorous, and vitamins A, B, C, and E.	Best when the tail is as long as the bean.
Millet, Unhulled Only	Jar or Bag	Long, 8-10	2	Serotonin and tryptophan regulate mood, appetite, sleep, muscle contraction, memory and learning. Also rich in anti-oxidants, magnesium (can help reduce the affects of migraines and heart attacks), niacin (can help lower cholesterol), phosphorus (helps with fat metabolism, tissue repair and energy production) and nutrients that protect against diabetes, cancer and asthma.	I've only ever been able to find unhulled online; see "resources" section.
Mung	Growing into bean sprouts is recommended, otherwise jar or bag	Long, 8-10	If sprouted by the rinse method, 2-4	Chlorophyll, iron, vitamin C, potassium, and are a complete protein	Watch out for duds if sprouting by the rinse method.

NAME	SPROUTING METHOD	SOAK TIME (HOURS)	SPROUT TIME/DAYS	NURIENTS/PROPERTIES	NOTES
Oats, Unhulled Only	Tray Method for Grass; Jar or Bag for Sprouts	Prolonged, 10-12 or more	2-3 for Sprouts; 6-9 for Grass	Amazing source of both kinds of fiber, a natural laxative, intestinal scrubber, and stool bulker. B vitamins, E, iron calcium, and GLA	The fibrousness of the husk varies a lot from company to company; less husk = less fiber but also less it has to be ground to break up the somewhat unpleasant tough fibers, which are like hard and sharp tiny strings in the mouth. See "Resources".
Pea	Jar or Bag for Sprouts; Tray Method for Pea Shoots	Prolonged, 10-12	1 day or more for Sprouts; for Pea Shoots 3-4 days covered or in the dark then 3-4 days in sun	Complex carbohydrates, calcium, magnesium, folic acid, vitamins A, Bs, C, and E. 25% protein. Green peas have chlorophyll.	Delicious and tender at any age. Will not get bitter so start a big batch and eat it for weeks. Huge variety of colors and sizes.
Peanut	Jar or Bag	Medium, 6-8	2, just after the point (the germ) has protruded	30% protein and 45% oil, very high in vitamin E, folate, niacin, riboflavin, magnesium, phosphorous, phytochemicals, and fiber.	A legume, not a nut, peanuts are an easy sprout and great way to bridge the mental gap between an inanimate everyday food and a growing seed.
Quinoa	Bag	Medium, 6-8	1-2	A complete protein, and higher in protein than any other grain. More calcium than milk and the cofactor magnesium, as well as silicon, iron, B vitamins, phosphorous and vitamin E, and magnesium, important in the fight against heart disease and diabetes. Manganese and copper fight the free radicals that cause cancer and aging.	A vital grain for a healthy population, fights heart disease, diabetes, and cancer, and could solve many of the world's biggest problems if it was the planet's primary protein source. Contains no gluten and is therefore not allergy-producing. High levels of enzyme inhibitors; change the soak water a couple of times. When rinsing, continue until there are no more foamy bubbles.
Rice, Brown	Germinated	Soaked 1 – 3 days		Fiber, GABA reduces anxiety and stress, magnesium, potassium, zinc, E and many B vitamins	Must be cooked. Improves health, digestibility and flavor, but is also a simple step that could lead to large-scale increase in food mass and amplified nutrition for much of the world.

NAME	SPROUTING METHOD	SOAK TIME (HOURS)	SPROUT TIME/DAYS	NURIENTS/PROPERTIES	NOTES
Rye	Tray Method for Grass; Jar or Bag for Sprouts	Prolonged – 10-12	2-3 for Sprouts; 6-9 for Grass	Fluorine strengthens teeth and tooth enamel, and its photoestrogenic lignans can help normalize hormone activity, helpful for all, especially the menopausal.	Less processed than whole wheat and retains more nutrients. Less gluten than wheat yield a dense, sweet-sour loaf. Grass juice is powerfully cleansing. Makes a sour-sweet probiotic water reminiscent of rye bread, pickles, and NY delis.
Sesame, Unhulled Only	Jar or Bag	Medium – 6-8	2	1000 times the calcium as milk, phosphorous, potassium, magnesium, and vitamin A.	Very easy to digest, rich oily flavor is great in both savory and sweet dishes, like hummus and halva, a sweet, dense confection popular in India, the Middle East, and North Africa.
Soybeans	Jar or Bag	2-12 depending on the seed; check every 2 hours for softness. Will fall apart if soaked too long.	2-5, depending on preference	A complete protein, also rich in iron, omega-3 fatty acids, tryptophan, molybdenum, manganese, fiber, vitamin K, magnesium, copper, B12 and potassium	Produces much more protein per acre than any other major vegetable crop, and much more than land used for meat or milk production. Can also rejuvenate nutrients in the soil. Sprouts are best ground, rinsed, and fermented.
Spelt	Tray Method for Grass; Jar or Bag for Sprouts	Prolonged – 10-12	2-3 for Sprouts; 6-9 for Grass	High in fiber, up to 25% more protein than wheat. Plentiful in B-vitamins, and special carbohydrates that assist in blood clotting and stimulating the immune system	Wheat's ancient ancestor. Not the best choice for grass juice, should be used in sprouted loaves that require a lighter, sweeter flavor than Kamut's butteriness.
Unhulled Sunflower, for Lettuce	Soil Method	Prolonged, 10-12	2-3 days covered with a wet towel, 5-7 days in the sun until the seeds mostly fall off, but before the second set of leaves come in.	Chlorophyll galore, all the vitamins and minerals below and more.	Will float insatiably in the soak water – submerge a filled sprout bag and weigh it down, or fill a jar until the seeds are high above the rim and screw on the lid, pushing all the seeds into the water.

NAME	SPROUTING METHOD	SOAK TIME (HOURS)	SPROUT TIME/DAYS	NURIENTS/PROPERTIES	NOTES
Sunflower Sprouts, Hulled	Jar or Bag	Medium, 6-8	1	33% protein, vitamins A, B complex, E, and D, and minerals including calcium, copper, iron, magnesium, potassium, phosphorus, and zinc. Omega-6 essential fatty acid. Phytosterols can help reduce cholesterol levels, lecithin is necessary to process EFAs and fats, both new and old. Tryptophan combats depression and stress.	Super easy sprout done before the first rinse. Can be therefore soaked with unsproutable nuts, like walnuts for an EFA balance, pumpkin seeds for a savory snack, or macadamias for a rich desserty treat. Won't sprout and will therefore lose a little nutrition if soaked in salt water, but won't trade their nutty flavor for a sprouty freshness – nice every once in a while.
Triticale	Tray Method for Grass; Jar or Bag for Sprouts	Prolonged, 10-12	2-3 for Sprouts; 6-9 for Grass		A combination of wheat and rye first bred by French botanists as a possible solution to world hunger as it's very quick and easy to grow, as well as rich in simple and complex carbohydrates.
Wheat	Tray Method for Grass; Jar or Bag for Sprouts	Prolonged, 10-12	2-3 for Sprouts; 6-9 for Grass		Use "hard red wheat berries" for grass juice. Good for grass and probiotic water (though not as good as Kamut, and not much cheaper or more available in an organic form.)
Wild Rice	Jar or Bag	Prolonged, 10-12	4-8	calcium, iron, magnesium, phosphorous, vitamins C, E, and B-6, is 15% protein.	Not rice nor grain, the fruit seed of a tall marsh grass enjoyed by Native Americans for the past 10 centuries. Will not grow a tail; is done which wild rice kernel split in two.
Herbs/Spices	Method	Soak, hours	Sprouting, Days	Flavor	Notes
Anise	Jar or Bag	Medium, 6-8	2	The true taste of licorice; digestive aid since Roman times.	

NAME	SPROUTING METHOD	SOAK TIME (HOURS)	SPROUT TIME/DAYS	NURIENTS/PROPERTIES	NOTES
Caraway	Jar or Bag	Medium, 6-8	2	Sweet, warming – pair with rye in probiotic water or sprouted bread for a robust deli flavor	
Cardamom	Jar or Bag	Prolonged, 24	3 – 6 weeks, if growing into a plant	Pungent and aromatic, with a eucalyptusy and lemony perfume, a digestive aid and and aphrodisiac	A seed pod with a thick hull, must be soaked and ground (preferable) or germinated
Celery	Jar or Bag for Sprouts, Basket for Nano Green Sprouts or Soil for Micro Greens	Medium, 6-8	2-3 for Sprouts: 5-9 for Micro Greens	Mild celery flavor is wonderful in many dishes	Very medicinal; can help fight cancer and cholesterol
Coriander	Jar or Bag, or Soil for Micro Cilantro	Medium, 6-8	2-3 for Sprouts, 5-9 for Micro Cilantro	Cooling and delicious	
Cumin	Jar or Bag	Medium, 6-8	2	Featured in Indian, Middle Eastern. and Latin cookery in both Europe and N. America	Many wonderful digestive benefits
Dill	Jar or Bag for Young Sprouts; Basket for Nano Greens	Medium, 6-8	2-3 for Young Sprouts; 5-9 for Nano Greens	Aromatic, fresh and slightly sweet flavor; equally at home in micro-green salads, spreads, and seed cheese	
Fennel	Jar or Bag for Young Sprouts; Basket for Nano Greens	Medium, 6-8	2-3 for Young Sprouts: 5-9 for Nano Greens	Warm, sweet and aromatic flavor similar to a mild anise.	Freshens the breath, suppresses appetite, digestive benefits; a wonderful addition to a salad mix.
Fenugreek	Jar or Bag	Long, 8-10	2-6 days; great very young or just after the first leaves show	Powerful, aromatic and bittersweet flavor; use in curries and with to balance very sweet tropical fruit, both in flavor and nutritionally.	Preferably yellow and tender; a quick sprout that doesn't need sun. Expectorant, anti-inflammatory, regulates blood sugar.
Garlic	Basket	Medium, 6-8	4-8	Garlicky! Easier on the stomach than raw garlic, but prohibitively slow and expensive.	Better to just plant some garlic in a yogurt container and cut its fast-growing tubular shoots as needed.

NAME	SPROUTING METHOD	SOAK TIME (HOURS)	SPROUT TIME/DAYS	NURIENTS/PROPERTIES	NOTES
Milk Thistle	Jar or Bag	Long, 8-10	1-2	Unparalleled liver cleanser and strengthener for better sleep, skin, and mood.	Hard-shelled; won't soften up much. Super bitter - best ground in juices in a high-speed blender, chewed up as a crunchy snack, or grond and put in capsules.
Mustard	Clay Planter Tray for Mucilages (Usually Brown): Jar or Bag for Dry (Usually Yellow)	Mucilage - Continous Soak. Dry Seed in Jar or Bag – Medium, 6-8	Long Soak – about 2, until a small tail protrudes, then refrigerate. Jar or Bag - 2-3	With a little apple cider vinegar, raw honey, and savory spices, makes a better mustard than you've ever had	Preferable yellow and tender, don't need sun. An emulsifier, go in almost all of my salad dressings and all soups and sauces inspired by Eastern European cuisines
Onion	Basket	Long, 8-10	4-8		Slow and expensive, better to use radish sprouts, or plant some green onion and cut its grass-like shoots
Poppy	Bag	Medium, 6-8	2 – will get bitter after	Not much flavor in small quantities so can be a versatile garnish; in larger quantities has a fresh and sweet taste, like candied bean sprouts.	Adds a beautiful metallic blue color to a dish when sprinkled on top.
Radish/Daikon	Basket for Micro Greens; Jar or Bag if with Salad Mix	Medium, 6-8	2-3 for Sprouts; 5-6 for Micro Greens	Spicy and zesty! Its heat is stimulating to the digestive system, removes mucous in the intestines and respiratory system, fires up elimination.	Will grow 16 times their size, so soak 1 T seeds for every 1 C. of sprouts. Move to a sunny spot after a couple day's growth. Antiseptic, anti-parasitic, and supportive to beneficial bacteria, so good for Candida sufferers (perhaps 85% of the population)

Appendix C:

Recommended Reading

Fermentation

Kitchen Sink Farming Volume 2: Fermenting by Jean-Pierre Parent

The Art of Fermentation: An In-Depth Exploration of Essential Concepts and Processes from Around the World by Sandor Ellix Katz and Michael Pollan

Wild Fermentation by Sandor Ellix Katz *with an incredible recommended reading list

Understanding: Bacteria Discovery Education School (DVD, and on youtube)

Sprouting:

Sprouts: The Miracle Food: The Complete Guide to Sprouting by Steve Meyerowitz and Michael Parman

The Sprouting Book: How to Grow and Use Sprouts to Maximize Your Health and Vitality by Ann Wigmore

The Wheatgrass Book: How to Grow and Use Wheatgrass to Maximize Your Health and Vitality by Ann Wigmore

Gardening:

Kitchen Sink Farming Volume 3: Growing by Jean-Pierre Parent

Fresh Food from Small Spaces: The Square-Inch Gardener's Guide to Year-Round Growing, Fermenting, and Sprouting by R.J. Ruppenthal

Dirt: the Ecstatic Skin of the Earth by William Bryant Logan

Vegetarianism, Veganism, and Raw Food Prep:

Kitchen Sink Farming Volume 4: What to Do with Your Sprouts and Krauts – Living Homegrown Recipes by Jean-Pierre Parent

Eating Animals by Jonathan Safran-Foer.

Diet for a New America and The Food Revolution by John Robbins.

Beyond Beef: The Rise and fall of the Cattle Culture by Jeremy Rifkin

RAW by Charlie Trotter

Ani's Raw Food Kitchen: Easy, Delectable Living Foods Recipes by Ani Phyo

Environment, GMOs, and Agribusiness:

The Power of Community: How Cuba Survived Peak Oil (DVD and on youtube)

The Weather of the Future by Heidi Cullen

Stolen Harvest: The Hijacking of the Global Food Supply by Dr. Vandana Shiva

The World According to Monsanto (DVD)

Evolution and Pleasure

Stumbling on Happiness by Daniel Gilbert

How Pleasure Works by Paul Bloom

Supernormal Stimuli: How Primal Urges Overran Their Evolutionary Purpose by Deidre Barrett

Practice Makes… Meditation and Yoga in Everyday Life by Jean-Pierre Parent

Appendix D:

Resources:

Seeds, Grains and Nuts:

NutsOnline.com - A family business with great prices, customer service, and a touch of whimsy in everything they do. They once sent a stuffed elephant with my order. Sold.

Wheatgrasskits.com - A great source for certain seeds as well as sprouting supplies.

Nutiva - The best hemp seeds and coconut oil. I get the 3-lb bag of organic shelled hempseeds and double pack of 54-oz jars of organic coconut oil. I buy them through amazon.com to get free shipping and a "Subscribe and Save" discount. They also make a raw coconut oil which comes in glass and is great, and more expensive.

Sprouting Bags – Available from great companies like Pure Joy Planet, but I use reusable mesh produce bags that are about 20 times cheaper and might last longer, but have a slightly wider mesh so the tiniest seeds like amaranth need the real deal. Or panty hose.

Probiotic Cultures

Dairy Kefir - kefirlady.com – a great source for dairy kefir grains grown in organic raw goat milk, and at the time of this writing she sells a ¼ cup for $20 with shipping; top-quality grains at the best price on the net for the quantity. She is also very available to answer questions and share the enthusiasm.

Kombucha, Juice Kefir, Apple Cider Vinegar – try your local craigslist first, then ebay. Can also be started from a raw, organic, and unflavored product from your local natural foods store.

Index

acetaminophen, 140
ADD, 61
Adzuki, 82
aging, 61, 91, 112, 119, 120
alcohol, 111, 146, 154
alfalfa, 52, 67, 72, 77, 83, 90, 91, 93
Alfalfa, 83
alkalinity, 110
Alkalinity, 111
alkaloids, 112, 150
allergies, 4, 58, 108, 118
allium, 149
almonds, 63, 98, 151, 153, 154, 155, 157
Alpha Linolenic Acid, 96
Alzheimer's, 125
amaranth, 70, 84, 174
Amaranth, 84
amasake, 125
Amazon, 118
amino acids, 8, 10, 54, 58, 61, 84, 90, 94, 100, 108, 120
ammonium nitrate, 31
Anheuser-Busch, 24
Anise, 137, 138
anti-coagulants, 129
anti-parasitic, 122
antiseptic, 122
antispasmodic, 138, 142
artheriosclerosis, 151
arthritis, 86, 140
artificial lighting, 56
arugula, 87
asthma, 110

Stay Connected!

Visit

www.KitchenSinkFarming.org

for tips, recipes, news, giveaways, and general delicious nerdiness.

Made in the USA
Coppell, TX
27 December 2019